CONTENTS

	Page
Introduction	1
Historical background	1
Taxonomy	2
Geographical distribution	4
Host range	5
Methods of detection	5
1. Smears of peripheral blood	5
2. Concentration of trypanosomes in peripheral blood	6
3. Culture	6
4. Serological diagnosis	9
Morphology	11
1. Morphology in peripheral blood	11
2. Morphology in tissues other than blood	15
3. Morphology in cultures	15
Cytochemistry	18
Pathogenicity	18
Immunology	21
Epidemiology	21
1. Geographical incidence	21
2. Age incidence	21
3. Levels of parasitaemia	22
4. The effect of chemotherapeutic agents	22
5. Natural transmission	23
6. Artificial transmission	27
Storage of strains	28
Life cycle	29
1. Stages in fixed tissues	29
2. Forms in peripheral blood	30
3. Transmission from mammalian host to a vector	30
4. Forms in an insect vector	30
5. Transmission from a vector to a susceptible host	32
Conclusions	32
Table 1	33
Table 2	37
Appendix	38
References	46

INFECTIONS OF CATTLE WITH TRYPANOSOMES OF THE SUBGENUS MEGATRYPANUM (HOARE 1964)

by

E. A. WELLS Ph.D MRCVS DTVM

Centre for Tropical Veterinary Medicine,
University of Edinburgh

Review Series No.10
of the
Commonwealth Bureau of Animal Health

COMMONWEALTH AGRICULTURAL BUREAUX

1972

First published in 1972
by the
Commonwealth Agricultural Bureaux
Farnham Royal, Slough SL2 3BN, England

Price £1.50

SBN 85198 253 0

Printed in Great Britain by
Unwin Brothers Limited
The Gresham Press, Old Woking, Surrey, England.

INTRODUCTION

Trypanosoma theileri Laveran, 1902 is recognized as a cosmopolitan parasite of domestic cattle (Herbert 1964) and represents the type species of the subgenus *Megatrypanum* in Hoare's classification of mammalian trypanosomes (Hoare 1966). Two other members of the subgenus have also been reported to infect cattle, *T. ingens* (Hamerton 1911; Mackie 1911; Panama 1941) and *T. tragelaphi* (Thomson 1931). Wenyon (1926) gives a list of other species names considered to be synonyms of *T. theileri*.

This review first describes the historical background to the discovery of these relatively large trypanosome species of mammals and then presents an argument in favour of calling all of these infections collectively '*T. theileri*-like'. The literature is then reviewed on this basis.

HISTORICAL BACKGROUND

The first recognition of a large trypanosome of cattle was probably made by Lingard in India in 1892, although he did not publish his observations until 1903. Legrain (1896) in France described a trypanosome found post-mortem in a pericardial haemorrhage of an ox and, later, Kossel & Weber recollected having seen a single large trypanosome in a heart muscle smear of an ox in Finland about 1900 (Schaudinn 1904; Weber 1909). However, Theiler (1903) was the first to attract major attention to a large trypanosome of cattle, because he believed at that time that it was the cause of an important cattle disease in South Africa known as 'galziekte' (gall sickness). He sent blood smears to both Laveran and Bruce, who independently suggested the species name *Trypanosoma theileri* in 1902. Laveran's paper took time precedence. Although Theiler later identified the disease as bovine anaplasmosis (Theiler 1910), much interest in the trypanosome was aroused, particularly when it was realized that the presence of similar organisms in peripheral blood of cattle, difficult to detect on direct microscopy, could be readily detected on culture (Miyajima 1907; Martini 1909; Crawley 1909). In the short period thereafter up to 1914 there are at least seventy published papers giving geographical localities in which large trypanosomes of either domestic or wild Bovidae were detected in peripheral blood either by direct microscopy or by culture. Other isolations were made in this period but not published, e.g. Steck in Switzerland (personal communication).

From the time of this intense interest to the present day few sustained studies exist, even though Johns (1914) suggested that such a large and easily obtainable trypanosome would be "very valuable to study the great problem of trypanosomiasis". The reasons for this have probably been, first, the failure to establish infection in any small laboratory animal and, second, the realization that the infection was normally non-pathogenic. John's view was, however, independently revived by the W. H. O. expert committee on immunology and parasitic diseases (W. H. O. 1965), who indicated a need for a model trypanosome available for "experimental, immunological and epidemiological study" in temperate climates and recommended that T. theileri be "intensively studied to determine its suitability for the purposes outlined".

TAXONOMY

The revised classification of the protozoa proposed by the committee on taxonomy and taxonomic problems of the Society of Protozoologists (Honigberg et al. 1964) places the genus Trypanosoma as follows:-

Phylum Protozoa Goldfuss, 1818; emend. Siebold, 1845
Subphylum Sarcomastigophora Honigberg & Balamuth, 1963
Superclass Mastigophora Diesing, 1866
Class Zoomastigophorea Calkins, 1909
Order Kinetoplastida Honigberg, 1963
Suborder Trypanosomatina Kent, 1880
Family Trypanosomatidae Doflein, 1901; emend. Grobben, 1905
Genus Trypanosoma Gruby, 1843.

The classification of members of the genus Trypanosoma offered by Wenyon (1926) was based on two main courses of development in the invertebrate host. The first is the development which leads to infection of the biting parts of the invertebrate with the metacyclic stage so that transmission can be termed 'inoculative', and the second is the development which leads to metacyclic forms in the hind gut so that transmission can be termed 'contaminative'. Wenyon therefore divided the genus into Group A, those trypanosomes which develop in the 'posterior station', and Group B, those trypanosomes which develop in the 'anterior station'. Hoare (1949, 1957), considering only the trypanosomes of mammals, classified them on this basis, giving additional reasons for the relevance of the grouping. He later proposed the terms "Stercoraria" and "Salivaria" in place of Groups A and B, subdividing both into four subgenera. T. theileri thus became the type species of the subgenus Megatrypanum (Hoare 1964). Hoare, in his latest modification (1966), states that the hosts of T. theileri are "bovines" and "antelopes", and places in the same subgenus the following selected species:-

Species	Author		Hosts
T. tragelaphi	Kinghorn et al.	(1913)	antelopes
T. melophagium	Flu	(1908)	sheep
T. mazamarum	Mazza et al.	(1932)	deer
T. cephalophi	Bruce et al.	(1915)	antelopes
T. ingens	Bruce et al.	(1909b)	cattle, antelopes, chevrotains

Hoare stated in his explanatory notes (1966), in reference to the Stercoraria, that "fuller studies of such species might necessitate a re-appraisal of their systematic position". This can be seen to be a possibility in the subgenus Megatrypanum, as amongst the selected species the vector is proven for T. melophagium alone (Hoare 1923) and the remainder are allocated on the evidence of hosts and morphology. Even evidence of the transmission of the type species is incomplete (see section: natural transmission).

The possible need for re-appraisal was further emphasized by Keymer (1967, 1969), who described trypanosomes identifiable on morphological grounds as T. theileri, T. cephalophi, T. tragelaphi and T. ingens, all in the same splenectomized ox in Malawi over a period of six weeks. He further believed that there was no obvious morphological difference "between any of the recognized species in the subgenus Megatrypanum". Davis (1952) met a similar difficulty with the trypanosomes of rodents (section Stercoraria, subgenus Herpetosome), and suggested the term "T. lewisi-like" for those isolations where only morphological data were available. "T. cruzi-like" trypanosomes has likewise become accepted phraseology in the Stercorarian subgenus Schizotrypanum (e.g. Deane 1967). Keymer (1967) therefore made the suggestion that T. cephalophi, T. tragelaphi and T. ingens should be referred to as "T. theileri-like" trypanosomes.

The assumption implicit in the W. H. O. recommendation that sufficient is known of the characteristics of Trypanosoma theileri to identify it as a valid and cosmopolitan species is seen to be open to discussion. For purposes of review, therefore, the species name Trypanosoma theileri is taken to refer only to Theiler's original observations in South Africa, and a list of T. theileri-like trypanosomes is made to absorb not only the list of synonyms of T. theileri offered by Wenyon (1926), but also the selected species of Hoare's 1966 classification, with the exception of T. melophagium. The list can then read:

Trypanosoma transvaaliense	Laveran	(1902b)
Trypanosoma lingardi	Blanchard	(1904)
Trypanosoma himalayanum	Lingard	(1907)
Trypanozoon theileri	Lühe	(1906)
Trypanosoma indicum	Lingard	(1907)
Trypanosoma muktesari	Lingard	(1907)
Trypanosoma brublewskii	Wladimiroff & Yakimoff	(1909)
Trypanosoma americanum	Crawley	(1909)
Trypanosoma franki	Frosch	(1909)
Trypanosoma falshawi	Knuth	(1909)
Trypanosoma scheini	Knuth	(1909)
Trypanosoma ingens	Bruce et al.	(1909b)
Trypanosoma rutherfordi	Hadwen (1912) quoted by Wenyon	(1926)
Trypanosoma cephalophi	Bruce et al.	(1913)
Trypanosoma schonebecki	Mayer	(1912)
Trypanosoma tragelaphi	Kinghorn et al.	(1913)
Trypanosoma theileri var. somalensis	Croverie	(1920)
Trypanosoma theileri var. soudanense	Curasson	(1925)
Trypanosoma mazamarum	Mazza et al.	(1932)

GEOGRAPHICAL DISTRIBUTION

Appendix 1 lists published and some unpublished records of the demonstration of T. theileri-like trypanosomes in mammalian tissues either by direct microscopy or by culture. Although not exhaustive, the list illustrates the cosmopolitan distribution of the organisms ranging from the tropics to the neighbourhood of the Arctic Circle. Relatively few references from some countries, for example Australia and China, and the total absence from others are likely to be due to lack of search. Admissions of failure to demonstrate the presence of the organisms in a country by means of culture techniques successful elsewhere are rare. Bettencourt & Borges (1912, 1916) failed to cultivate trypanosomes from approximately 50 head of cattle arriving in Portugal from the Azores, whereas infections were easily detected on the Portuguese mainland.

HOST RANGE

Records of trypanosomes of the subgenus Megatrypanum are all derived from animals of the mammalian Order Artiodactyla (even-toed ungulates). Records of T. theileri-like trypanosomes in particular relate either to the domestic ox (Bos taurus) or to the domestic zebu (Bos indicus) (family Bovidae, subfamily Bovinae). As authors often fail to state which of these two species is involved, no distinction will be made in this review, and both will be referred to as cattle.

All records of T. theileri-like trypanosomes seen in blood smears made from other artiodactyl species are consolidated in Table 1. They overwhelmingly relate to the family Bovidae but this distribution of records may be misleading, for two reasons. First, most records have been incidental to a search in Africa for silent hosts of the salivarian trypanosomes pathogenic to man or his domestic animals. This has resulted in uneven sampling within the order, with particular neglect of the 41 species representing the family Cervidae. Stercorarian trypanosome parasitaemias of domestic cattle are normally submicroscopic and are only detected on blood agar culture media. Similar levels of parasitaemia may be present in other artiodactyls, but only a few culture attempts have been made (Table 2).

Wells (1969) listed 68 recorded, unsuccessful attempts by various workers to infect sheep and goats, representatives of other mammalian orders, and birds, using blood or cultures from domestic cattle known to be infected with T. theileri-like trypanosomes. Curasson (1925, 1943), however, claimed to have transmitted T. theileri-like trypanosomes of cattle to sheep and goats and to have demonstrated transient infections, and Vrijburg (1912) claimed to have induced a transient infection in a horse (Order Perissodactyla). Although transmission experiments have been tentative and there has been this one claim of success in a representative of another mammalian order, the impression is confirmed that trypanosomes of the subgenus Megatrypanum are restricted in their host range to members of the Order Artiodactyla.

METHODS OF DETECTION

1. Smears of peripheral blood

Levels of parasitaemia with T. theileri-like infections of cattle are normally too low to allow diagnosis from smears. They may be seen, however, on rare occasions wherever experiments are carried out involving either the repeated examination of the blood of an ox for haemoparasites, e.g. Saisawa et al. (1933) in Japan and Atchley (1951) in the U.S.A., or routine blood counts (Benbrook & Sloss 1961). More information comes from countries where diagnostic services routinely examine large numbers of blood smears from cattle. In Uganda, for example, (Uganda: Annual Reports, Department of Veterinary Services), out of a total of 68,674 blood smears examined for haemoparasites in 22 years, 630 showed one or more T. theileri-like trypanosomes (0.92%).

Information on the ease of blood smear diagnosis in other artiodactyls is too scanty for comparison. Whereas Reid et al. (1966) showed that submicroscopic parasitaemias can exist in the bushbuck (Tragelaphus scriptus), Keymer (1969) found T. (Megatrypanum) spp. on blood slides of 46 out of 95 duiker (Sylvicarpra grimmia) shot in Malawi, Zambia and Rhodesia.

2. Concentration of trypanosomes in peripheral blood

The concentration of trypanosomes in the peripheral blood has been attempted by centrifuging whole blood and examining the leucocyte layer for trypanosomes (e.g. Miyajima 1907; Crawley 1912b; Johns 1913, 1914). Other authors centrifuged blood after haemolysing with an equal volume of distilled water (e.g. Teague & Clark 1918; Turner & Murname 1930a, b; Saisawa et al. 1933). None of these authors had consistent success. The haematocrit centrifuge method used by Woo (1969) for T. pipientis of the frog has an obvious application. Likewise the DEAE-cellulose column (Lanham 1968, 1970) has not been used for T. theileri-like trypanosomes, although the method has been applied to other stercorarian infections of mammals.

3. Culture

T. theileri-like trypanosomes may be cultured both at temperatures experienced by a vector and at the temperature of a mammalian host.

a. Culture at vector temperature. A single reference records active division of trypanosomes in parasitaemic peripheral blood withdrawn from an ox. Crawley (1912b) centrifuged peripheral blood from an ox 4 hours after withdrawal and found clumps of flagellates, probably in active division. Robinson (1923) claimed that growth could be obtained to a level of microscopic diagnosis by the simple addition of an isotonic dextrose solution (5.4% in distilled water). The majority of prepared media used have either been variations of "bouillon" (e.g. Miyajima 1907; Martini 1909; Crawley 1909, 1912b) or variations of rabbit blood-agar slopes introduced by Novy & MacNeal (1904) for the cultivation of Trypanosoma brucei. Examples of both types provide efficient isolation media, but some authors noticed that subculture was only possible on blood agar (e.g. Delanoe 1911; Manceaux et al. 1911a; Kohl-Yakimoff et al. 1913a). The observation by Nöller (1917, 1931) that the enriching of the agar component with nutrient broth enabled indefinite subculture was confirmed by Herbert (1962, 1965b), who also showed that the mammalian blood component should represent a minimum of 20% of the medium. Horse, ox, sheep, goat, dog and rabbit blood were successfully used by Trautmann (1922), but Herbert (1965b) demonstrated that many samples of human blood and some samples of ox blood were unsuitable.

Herbert made a particular study of a continuously subcultured strain of trypanosome which he obtained from Eire and termed Trypanosoma theileri (1965c). He showed that it "grew well under conditions of aerobiosis, anaerobiosis and reduced oxygen tension. Cultures of T. theileri were depressed in vitro by the presence of tissue products of culture metabolism and of a low pH; they were also depressed when culture medium was inoculated with trypanosomes passaged from a declining culture". No growth was obtained on blood-free media despite many attempts, although growth became possible when such media were separated from defibrinated blood by a semipermeable membrane.

In relation to the characteristics of primary isolation, Crawley (1912b) commented that infections were more difficult to detect on culture in winter than in summer, and that "autumn" cultures required on the average a significantly longer period of incubation than isolations made in the "spring" and "summer". Reports of the longevity of primary cultures vary widely. Using bouillon type media, Carpano (1913) reported only 20 days of life, while Vrijburg (1912) reported 120 days. Herbert (1965a) ceased counting cultures on blood agar at day 23 as "the organisms had declined in number and were no longer clearly staining due to the protein precipitation that accumulates in the culture vessel.....". Nöller (1917) believed that his test-tube blood-agar cultures died out in about 30 days, but recorded having occasionally seen "lively, motile, flagellum bearing forms" on plate cultures at day 47, together with "rounded off vacuolated degenerate forms". Packchanian (1943) found "occasional" cultures still motile at day 120. Wells (1971b) examined all these phenomena in relation to infected cattle in Scotland, and found that levels of parasitaemia, required length of incubation and longevity of primary isolations all varied seasonally. This is later discussed in relation to the life-cycle of T. theileri-like trypanosomes.

T. theileri-like trypanosomes have been accidentally cultured from peripheral blood of cattle in Europe in the course of other investigations (e.g. Kerr & Robertson 1943) and may be only of incidental interest. In Africa, however, they may complicate the diagnosis on culture of important salivarian trypanosomes. Bolton (1965 - personal communication) obtained cultures of T. theileri-like flagellates on a diphasic medium which supported T. congolense, and Gray & Nixon (1967) used for their T. theileri investigations a medium originally developed for T. rhodesiense and T. gambiense (Tobie et al. 1950).

Unawareness of the universal distribution of T. theileri-like trypanosomes has led some workers into errors of diagnosis. Novy & MacNeal (1904) obtained flagellates on culture from an ox in the Philippines and assumed that they had cultured T. evansi. Bruce et al. (1909a) accepted the assumption, but Gaiger (1910) pointed out that the flagellates could have been T. theileri. A similar error was probably made by Bruce when he reported the culture of T. vivax (Bruce et al. 1910).

b. Culture at mammalian host temperature. Attempts to grow T. theileri-like trypanosomes at mammalian blood temperatures can be divided into four groups. The first group consists of the attempts to raise the temperature of cultures first established at room temperature on "bouillon" or blood agar media, the second group contains attempts to develop other blood-containing media for use specifically at mammalian blood temperatures, the third group contains attempts to grow trypanosomes on cultures of other mammalian tissues in the total absence of red blood cells, and the last group is growth on chick embryos.

In the first group the common experience has been that cultures established at room temperature die when the temperature is raised to 37° C. Robinson (1923), for example, found no development in broth culture at the higher temperature after 3 days, and Glaser (1922) and Herbert (1964) found survival times of 3 - 5 days and 2 - 5 days, respectively, on blood agar slopes. Trautmann (1922) appears to be the only worker who has described the occasional growth of these organisms on a blood agar medium at 35° C with change of morphology to the trypomastigote form associated with the mammalian host. If Trautmann used the same medium constituents as Nöller (1916), this may be of some significance, as his plates would have contained 50% whole blood, as compared to the more usual 25%.

In the second group, Ristic & Trager (1958) recorded a successful attempt to isolate T. theileri–like organism on a medium maintained at 37° C. They used a mixture of lysed ox red blood cells in homologous serum, whole blood from the same animal, and glucose, to which was added whole blood from the animal to be tested. Simpson & Green (1959) also successfully utilized bovine haemolysate, but only as a small addition to trypticase soy broth. Herbert (1965c), however, did not have the same success with these media using his trypanosome strain isolated from Eire which had been continuously subcultured on blood agar. Splitter & Soulsby (1967) had noted that T. theileri in trypomastigote form had been reported as a contaminant of tissue cultures, and therefore studied the usefulness of three commercially available tissue culture fluids as media components for the production of large numbers of the organism for immunological studies. The three tissue culture fluids were also evaluated in combination with veal infusion broth or trypticase soy broth. Failure to passage never occurred if red blood cells were included in the medium or replaced with bovine blood coagulum, but, like Herbert, they had little success with haemolysate. As a development of this work Sollod & Soulsby (1968) modified an initial culture medium over a series of 51 subcultures in a period of one year and succeeded in growing the organisms in a final ambient containing haemin and a defined modification of McCoy 5a tissue culture medium. They claimed therefore that Trypanosoma theileri had become the first mammalian trypanosome to be serially cultured in a medium free from blood and cells at 37° C.

In relation to the third group of culture attempts, growth on cultures of mammalian tissues appears first to have been noted as a contamination of cultures prepared for other purposes. Examples are Lundholm et al. (1959) for contamination of a bovine foetal kidney cell culture, Malmquist (1965) for lymph node cells, and Cross et al. (1968) for contamination of a buffy coat culture. It can be supposed that many unpublished observations exist. Van Der Maaten & Malmquist (1969) discussed how these trypanosome contaminants of bovine cell cultures might be removed. The contamination of mammalian cell cultures has helped to prompt more specific studies. Lundholm et al. (1959) thus also observed that trypanosomes could multiply in the absence of cells in tissue culture media containing 10% by volume lamb serum, but multiplication appeared more rapid when tissue culture cells were present.

Wells (1971a) inoculated six isolates of T. theileri-like organisms derived from Scotland onto cultures of leucocytes on separate occasions. On three occasions he found the organisms adhering to the monolayer by their posterior ends as single organisms, occasionally in division, within 24 hours. On the other three occasions, the organisms were found in active division in colonies by 24 hours and were not found adhering to the monolayer until examination at 48 or 72 hours. Other specific studies were made by Hare & Soulsby (1969) on the "stimulation of DNA synthesis in bovine leucocyte cultures by Trypanosoma theileri antigens", following suggestions made in discussion by Hare et al. (1967) and Yang et al. (1967). Their studies were preliminary, but indicated that the peripheral blood mononuclear leucocytes of some cattle are capable of responding in vitro to an antigen prepared from T. theileri.

Lastly, only Woo et al. (1970) appear to have grown T. theilieri-like trypanosomes on chick embryos at 37° C after preliminary isolation from cattle on a blood agar medium at 26 - 28° C.

The ease with which T. theileri-like trypanosome isolations can be made from the field and transferred from media at room temperature to media at mammalian blood temperature indicates a system readily available both for teaching demonstration and further investigation.

4. Serological diagnosis

The information available is of a very miscellaneous nature, and a method of serological diagnosis has not been standardized.

Theiler (1903) described agglutination of Trypanosoma theileri in defibrinated blood, but there might have been confusion with the rosette appearance of actively multiplying trypanosome colonies. Gray & Nixon (1967) specifically stated that suspensions of T. theileri-like flagellates from cultures were unsuitable for use as antigens in agglutination tests, as the organisms were growing in firm clumps when harvested.

Nevertheless, Trautmann (1922), summarized by Mesnil (1923), used an agglutination test to show that the serum of infected cattle, as that of the horse, sheep, goat and dog, agglutinated T. theileri-like trypanosomes at dilutions of 1:10 to 1:80. The diluted sera, if not activated, were trypanocidal. By inference, from Mesnil's summary, Trautmann used culture forms obtained from blood agar plates maintained at room temperature. The antigenic relationship between forms on culture at room temperature and forms in peripheral blood requires to be established, together with their relationship to similar populations of other trypanosome species. This consideration applies to both the work of Robinson (1923) and that of Gray & Nixon (1967).

Robinson attempted to make an antigen from room temperature cultures for use in a complement fixation test to detect the pathogenic trypanosome infections of domestic animals in South Africa. No reactions were observed. Gray & Nixon used an antigen consisting of homogenized blood agar culture forms, and failed to show precipitin reactions with serum from cattle infected with T. theileri-like organisms. However, they also found that none of the serum samples from the infected cattle reacted with antigens of Trypanosoma vivax and T. brucei in agglutination and precipitin tests, and had no difficulty in infecting cattle, which carried infections with T. theileri-like organisms, with T. congolense and T. vivax in laboratory studies. They concluded that infections with T. theileri-like organisms are unlikely to be of practical importance in immunological studies of infections with pathogenic trypanosomes based on agglutination and precipitin reactions. Schoening (1925) also failed to reveal any cross reactions between T. equiperdum and T. theileri-like organisms. He cultured the latter organisms from 17 of 26 cattle, but none of the cattle were serologically positive to a complement fixation test using T. equiperdum as antigen.

Splitter et al. (1967) alone have attempted serological work with T. theileri-like organisms grown at 37° C. They found precipitins present "in the sera of 10 of 17 cattle naturally infected with T. theileri, but the indirect haemagglutination test appeared to be of little or no value in detecting T. theileri antibodies, even in cattle whose sera showed precipitin reactions with the T. theileri antigen". The antigen was harvested from culture at about the sixth day, when approximately 60 - 70% of flagellates were in the trypomastigote form (Splitter & Soulsby 1967). The possibility remains, therefore, that precipitation techniques will be limited in their application to pathogenic trypanosomes if cross-reaction occurs with T. theileri-like organisms. No work, however, has been done with an antigen prepared from flagellates grown on mammalian tissue culture.

Onyango (1967), reporting on an indirect fluorescent antibody test for bovine tsetse-transmitted trypanosomiasis, described preliminary work to provide a base line for fluorescence. Cattle infected and not infected with T. theileri-like organisms were compared, and serum samples taken from infected herds were found to be more reactive.

No clear answer appears to be available to the question whether T. theileri-like organisms can interfere with the serological diagnosis of salivarian trypanosomes.

MORPHOLOGY

1. Morphology in peripheral blood (fig. 1)

Wide variations occur in the descriptions of T. theileri-like flagellates under the light microscope. However, in some instances, authors have not clearly stated whether the flagellum has or has not been included in the length of the organism, and often the methods used to fix and stain preparations have not been mentioned when these may significantly alter the size of the flagellates (see Walker 1963). The thickness of a preparation can also alter apparent width of a large trypanosome (Keymer 1969). Detailed comparisons of the copious and meticulous measurements recorded by early workers, e.g. Lingard (1907), are therefore unjustified, excepting to note the order of size in terms of length and width and in the relative position of the organelles.

Laveran (1902a, b) examined blood slides sent to him by Theiler, and described Trypanosoma theileri as a trypanosome varying in length from 30 to 60 μ (including flagellum) and in width from 2 to 4 μ. He further described a slender, pointed, posterior end, a centrally placed nucleus, a deeply staining kinetoplast at the posterior end, a free flagellum one quarter of the total length and a finely granular protoplasm. He claimed, however (1902b), that he identified a second trypanosome species in further slides sent to him, which he called T. transvaaliense. This species varied from T. theileri in being 18 - 50 μ long (including flagellum), but principally in that the kinetoplast was always near or even attached to the nucleus (epimastigote form; Hoare & Wallace 1966). Theiler himself (1903) disagreed with this view and believed that T. transvaaliense was merely a development form of T. theileri of greater width, and comparatively rare. He considered that longitudinal division could occur in both forms, but that in the T. transvaaliense type the kinetoplast moved adjacent to the nucleus before division commenced. Subsequent observers have not challenged the shape and arrangements of the trypomastigote form as described by Laveran (1902a), and their comments are discussed here in terms of range of size of trypomastigote forms, the epimastigote form in relation to the division of the parasite, and motility in wet preparations.

Most authors have inferred that trypomastigote forms seen in peripheral blood can be placed in distinct groups as, for example, the "long slender" and "short thick" forms of Lühs (1905) or the "large narrow", "large wide" and "small slender" forms of Behn (1912) and Bonger (1913). Woo et al. (1970) found trypanosomes of two ranges of

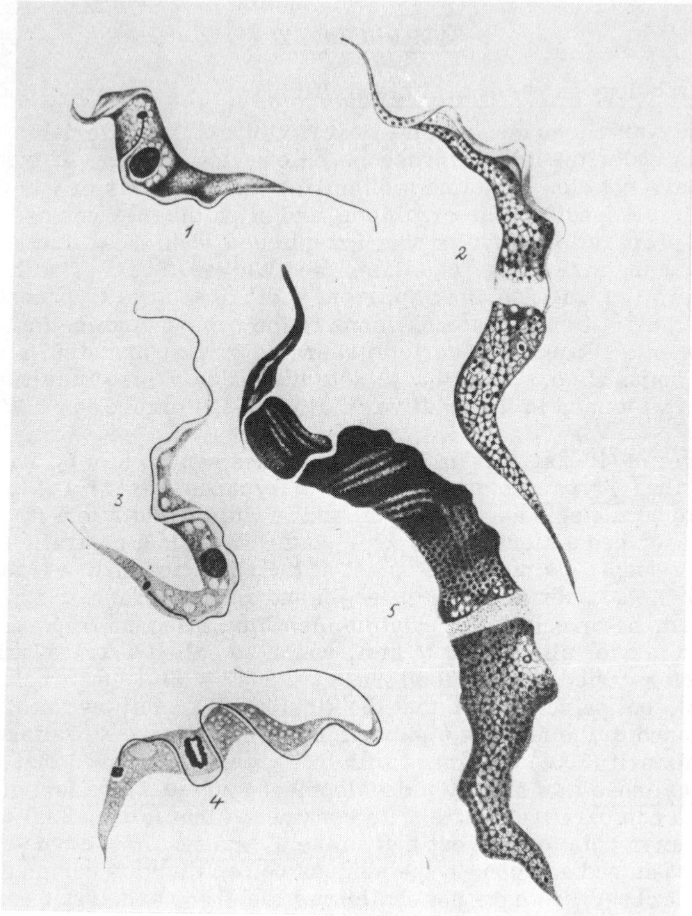

Figure 1. Large trypanosomes of mammals (x2000). A composite illustration after Wenyon (1926) from published material by Bruce et al. (1915) (1), Bruce et al. (1910) (5), Kinghorn & York (1913) (2), Lühe (1906) (3 and 4). (1) Trypanosoma cephalophi (2) T. tragelaphi (3) and (4) T. theileri (5) T. ingens.

body length in five cattle in Ontario, Canada. They had ranges of 22.7 - 40.7 μ and 8.29 - 13.30 μ, respectively. The authors considered the larger trypanosomes to be T. theileri and the smaller to be another species which they considered to be T. uniforme-like (Section Salivaria). Both populations could be identified on blood smears from the five cattle, and both could be grown in a blood agar medium and on chick embryos. Other authors have concluded that size is related to the stage of infection in the host, the largest sizes being associated with older infections (Teague & Clark 1918; Reichenow 1940; Touré 1968). The observation by Wells (1971a) that trypanosomes growing on leucocyte cultures increase in size with age of culture may be pertinent information in this respect. Keymer (1969) plotted a frequency distribution curve of the body length measurements of T. theileri-like trypanosomes from a variety of sources. He found that the curve for the "grand total of 314 measurements shows a normal length distribution ranging from 10 μ to 130 μ". Moreover, as already described (see section: taxonomy), he saw parasites identifiable from Hoare's classification (1966) as T. theileri, T. cephalophi, T. tragelaphi and T. ingens in the same splenectomized ox over a period of six weeks.

Relatively few authors have described forms in division occurring in peripheral blood. Lühs (1905) agreed with Theiler's interpretation of the epimastigote forms as being a stage prior to division. He described longitudinal division resulting in daughter trypanosomes of equal size and transverse division resulting in daughters of unequal size. Carpano (1913, 1924) also stated that the epimastigote form occurred at the time of division of the organism when the posterior end also rounded off. Reichenow (1940) described binary division as characteristically resulting in unequal daughter cells, and in the smaller of these the kinetoplast was initially adjacent to the nucleus, but later moved posteriorly. These short forms continued to multiply and the long forms were in transition to giant forms of "chronic" infections. The illustrations of Lühs (1905) and Reichenow (1940) are compared in figure 2. Other authors reported epimastigote forms, but offered no opinions of their significance (Schein 1907; Haughwout & Youngberg 1920; Glaser 1922; Curasson 1925; Tendeiro 1949).

Descriptions of motility of blood forms have varied widely. Flagella have been described as actively lashing but with little or no translatory movement of the parasites (e.g. Stockman 1910; Johns 1913; Hornby et al. 1934), while other accounts refer to rapid translatory movement (e.g. Schein 1907; Carpano 1913; Croverie 1920). Some authors describe a capability of the trypanosomes to attach by their posterior ends to leucocytes (Johns 1913), red blood cells (Lühs 1905) or to the glass slide (Hornby & Bailey 1929).

In summary, therefore, T. theileri-like trypanosomes seen in the peripheral blood of hosts show a wide variation in body length probably extending from 10 to 130 μ, commonly in the trypomastigote form but

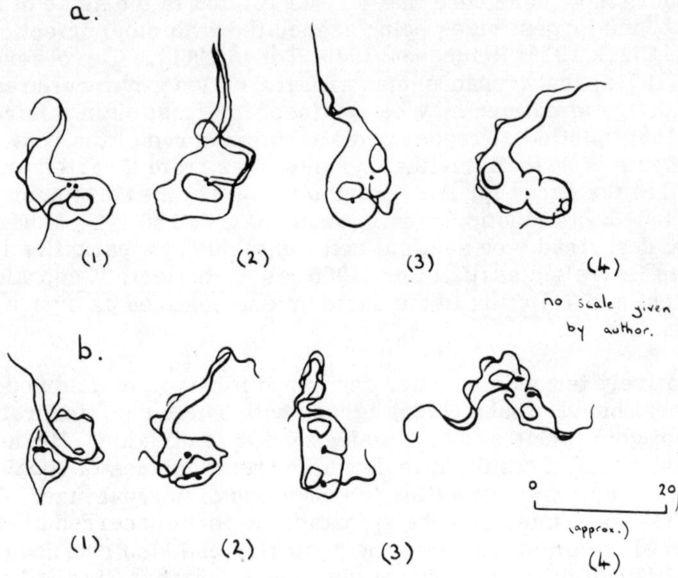

Figure 2. Unequal division of T. theileri-like trypanosomes in the peripheral blood. Drawings taken from the illustratsions of (a) Lühs (1905) and (b) Reichenow (1940).

occasionally epimastigote. The observations on variation in size, including those of Woo et al. (1970), may represent different stages in the life cycle of these organisms, and lack of realization of their occurrence could have assisted the proliferation of species names at the beginning of the present century.

2. Morphology in tissues other than blood

Sudachenkov (1931) found "large trypanosomes" in ulcerations of the bladder of a cow with haematuria, but the principle evidence of T. theileri-like trypanosomes multiplying in tissues other than blood relates to lymph nodes and the brain. Carpano (1932) found T. theileri-like organisms in a hypertrophied bovine prescapular lymph node. He described: amastigote forms smaller than bovine red blood cells; rounded "plasmodial" forms exceeding 15 μ in diameter with possibly more than one nucleus but each accompanied by a kinetoplast; promastigote forms of only 5 - 7 μ with the flagellum either extending externally or twisting internally; epimastigote forms 10 - 40 μ long including flagellum, identical to those which may be found in peripheral blood or in culture of blood at room temperature; and lastly a few trypomastigote forms 50 - 60 μ long including flagellum which correspond to those found in circulating blood. Gallo (1938) gave a similar description from lymph nodes of cattle with haemorrhagic septicaemia (pasteurellosis), but did not see trypomastigote forms. Croverie (1920), on the other hand, stated that the T. theileri-like organism which he studied was never encountered in lymph nodes.

Carpano (1932) and Gallo (1938) also described the amastigote, promastigote, epimastigote and trypomastigote forms in brain lesions. Carpano described the lesion as an area of haemorrhagic softening, and Gallo as a centre of degeneration. Carmichael (1939) found T. theileri-like organisms in the brain of an ox which had died from "turning sickness". He described the brain lesion as a "roughly circular patch of haemorrhagic softening about the size of a walnut with a tendency to necrosis". In smears and sections, however, he found only amastigote and epimastigote forms in large numbers. Barnett (1947) found similar lesions in another animal which had died from "turning sickness". In recollection (1966 - personal communication) the brain had several foci of 1/2 - 2 cm. diameter, especially in the cerebrum. These consisted of a semi-liquid necrotic centre with haemorrhagic periphery. The organisms present in the lesions were "shorter in length" than the trypomastigote forms of T. theileri found in peripheral blood.

3. Morphology in cultures

a. Cultures at room temperatures. Many descriptions are available of the morphology of T. theileri-like trypanosomes, both in liquid and in diphasic media. Some variations within the wide range of possibilities described may be entirely attributable to the constituents of the medium used (Carpano 1938), but comparison of descriptions of primary isolations of T. theileri-like trypanosomes in different media reveals the common appearance of certain morphological types. These are clearly described by Crawley (1912b), who used a beef bouillon medium (see fig. 3).

In wet preparations of 2 - 3 day old cultures Crawley saw both "broad" and "slender" flagellates as solitary organisms, in pairs, or in clusters of a few organisms. By 3 - 4 days the clusters could be relatively large, composed principally of long, slender, "band"-shaped organisms and others of a "club" form, the head of the club bearing the flagellum. By 5 - 6 days there were both large and small clusters with a greater number of free individuals. These, however, were not only of the "band" or "club" shapes, but also oval and short. Any or all of these forms could be found in division. Crawley was of the opinion that the sequence of development started with the short, "broad" form followed by the "band" and "club" shapes. The narrow posterior end of the "clubs" then reduced to a spike forming finally the oval shape. In old cultures (63 days) Crawley described masses of feebly motile round forms.

Crawley's observations on fixed and stained material gave flagellates at 4 - 5 days of culture growth a maximum body length of approximately 25 μ. At 10 days the maximum body length approximated 38 μ, with the length of the flagellum appearing to increase with the age of the culture. All forms were epimastigote in that the kinetoplast was invariably adjacent to the nucleus, and most often anteriorly. His description of a terminal flagellar knob or thickening has been confirmed by many authors in their drawings or photographs, if not in their text.

Crawley (1909, 1912b) in addition gave a clear description of the movement of the flagella in young cultures. Most movements were confined to vigorous lashings of the flagella, and the "club" forms showed a quick jerking with a shift in position of the long axis. A few forms showed rapid progressive movement. No author appears to surmise whether these latter minority have any distinctive morphology or are related to the very motile forms seen by Nöller (1917) in an old culture.

Crawley did not, however, record the trypomastigote forms in culture described by Delanoe (1911), Manceaux et al. (1911a, b), Herbert (1965a) and Touré (1968), nor promastigote forms (Herbert 1965a), although the latter may be equivalent to his epimastigote forms where the kinetoplast is anterior to the nucleus. In addition his "masses" of round forms in old cultures are usually illustrated or described as individuals e. g. Yakimoff & Schokor (1916). The detailed cytological study of Hartmann & Nöller (1918) did not mention or illustrate a "club" form. Their cultures were derived from flagellates infecting Tabanus glaucopis, but were said by Trautmann (1922) to be similar to cultures obtained from the peripheral blood of cattle. There appears to be no clear explanation.

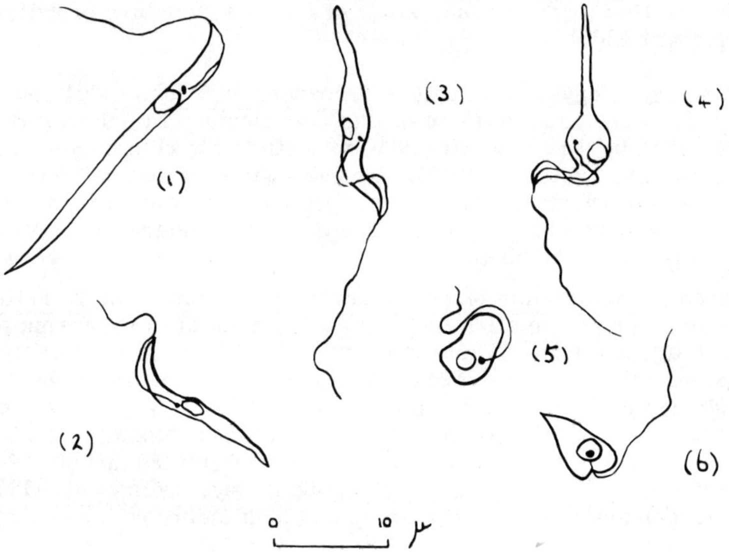

Figure 3. The morphology of T. theileri-like trypanosomes on culture at room temperatures. Drawings taken from the illustrations of Crawley (1909).

Herbert (1965a) related changes in morphology on culture to different stages of population growth, and associated "globular" forms (the "club" and "oval" forms of Crawley) with the population decline. This change in morphology was associated with an increasing number and size of cytoplasmic inclusions, and Herbert believed that the changes were comparable to those described as "degenerative" by Blacklock (1912) for T. rhodesiense and T. gambiense in the carcass of an animal host. He has also made the only study of the fine structure of culture forms (Herbert 1965b).

The morphology of the alleged Trypanosoma wrublewskii requires mention. The epimastigote form of this trypanosome in peripheral blood described by Wrublewskii (1909) was similarly commented upon by Mesnil (1913) and Yakimoff (1915). Mesnil suggested that as blood was collected from dead animals and then kept in a pipette for a number of days, the form seen was as if in culture at room temperature. A knobbed flagellum was also described.

b. Cultures at mammalian blood temperatures. Culture of T. theileri-like organisms on mammalian tissue cultures results in the formation of trypomastigote forms. There appear to be no figures on their proportion, excepting that Hulliger (1964 - personal communication) observed only "few" epimastigote forms. Splitter & Soulsby (1967), using their tissue culture media reinforced with broth and whole blood, found 30 - 40% of epimastigote forms at up to 6 days of culture and 60 - 70% epimastigote forms between the sixth and tenth day. Woo et al. (1970) saw only trypomastigote forms growing on chick embryos.

CYTOCHEMISTRY

Herbert (1965a) examined the cytochemistry of a T. theileri-like trypanosome, using his strain serially passaged on a blood agar medium (Herbert 1961). Newton (1971) separated three DNA components of T. theileri-like trypanosomes and found that the differences between strains isolated in Ayr (Scotland) and Bogotá (Colombia) were significant and reproducible.

PATHOGENICITY

Theiler (1903) at first claimed that Trypanosoma theileri was the cause of "gall sickness", an important cattle disease in South Africa, but later retracted this statement (1910), identifying the disease as anaplasmosis. The common belief since that time has been that T. theileri-like organisms have no pathogenic significance, but acute and sometimes fatal clinical episodes have been described in relation to their presence. These can be considered firstly in situations where the trypanosome is the only recognized infection, and secondly where the trypanosome occurs as a mixed infection with one or more pathogens.

T. theileri-like organisms have been reported in focal lesions in the brain, causing acute nervous symptoms (Carpano 1932; Gallo 1938; Carmichael 1939; Barnett 1947). Accounts also exist of T. theileri-like organisms found in large numbers in the peripheral blood of cattle which had died suddenly e.g. Frank (1909) and Kränzle (1912) in Germany, Sassouchin & Matwejeff (1922, quoted by Sprinholz-Schmidt 1938) and Berezin (1930) in Russia, Robinson (1923) in South Africa, and Wyssman (1935) and Bourgeois (1941) in Switzerland. Frosch (1909) believed that Frank had described a new trypanosomal disease, and made careful investigation of other cattle in the neighbourhood of the occurrence. Mayer (1909) disbelieved this conclusion, but Frank & Frosch (1909) stated that trypanosomiasis must be borne in mind when cases of anthrax were being investigated, a view continued to be held in 1938 by Schmid and independently by Vrijburg.

Other clinical episodes associated with the presence of T. theileri-like organisms alone are miscellaneous in character: Valladares (1909) described an acute fatal syndrome in an ox associated with swollen legs and urticarial eruptions on the chest; Sudachenkov (1931) saw the trypanosomes in ulcerations of the bladder of a cow with haematuria; Hall (1953) described a Canadian episode where 20 cattle died out of 45, but the reference contains no identification of the trypanosome concerned or the grounds for diagnosis; Levine et al. (1956) found T. theileri-like trypanosomes in blood smears of a heifer which had exhibited abortion, diarrhoea, and depression over a three month period; Dikmans et al. (1957) found the trypanosomes in the stomach contents of an aborted calf; Ristic & Trager (1958) cultivated the trypanosomes from three cows with depressed milk production and eosinophilia; an anonymous contribution to the Communicable Disease Centre, veterinary public health notes (1966) reported parasitaemias associated with a profuse diarrhoea and watery blood in six new-born calves, the dams having had high temperatures at the time of parturition; Lamy & Bouley (1967) found a heavy parasitaemia in a calf born at full term in a comatose state. The calf died the same day.

Most reports of T. theileri-like trypanosomes in relation to disease have been in association with concurrent infections with agents of recognized pathogenicity. Wells (1969) listed 57 such references in relation to ten bacterial, viral or protozoal diseases. Only in relation to rinderpest is there any allegation that these trypanosomes can aggravate the course of an infection. The evidence can be discussed first in terms of general observations from the field, and secondly in relation to circumstances where it is likely that rinderpest virus and T. theileri-like trypanosomes were inoculated simultaneously into experimental animals.

From the field, Theiler (1903), Lühs (1905) and Carpano (1913) independently commented that T. theileri-like parasitaemias were very common in association with rinderpest; Holmes (1904) believed that such parasitaemias occurred secondarily to an attack of rinderpest; Curasson (1925) detected a parasitaemia in a "latent" attack of the disease; Kearney (1926) reported that T. theileri was the trypanosome most frequently seen in Northern Nigeria in 1925, but added that the cattle examined were also infected with rinderpest, a fact enlarged upon by Glover (1961) who re-examined the records. Lastly, Croverie (1920) stated that the trypanosome appreciably modified the character of the disease.

Most information, however, has come from the "double inoculation" method of immunizing cattle against rinderpest which involved passaging the virus through cattle to obtain immune serum from recovered animals. A temperature reaction normally followed the inoculation of viraemic blood. In some cases, after an interval of some days, a second temperature rise could be observed, associated with a high parasitaemia with T. theileri-like trypanosomes. At this second temperature rise death could occur. This phenomenon was reported many times from many countries, e.g. Theiler (1903), Holmes (1904), Durrant & Holmes (1904), Schein (1907), Robertson (1956), Haughwout & Youngberg (1920), Carmichael (1926), and Hornby et al. (1934). Other relevant information is provided by Lühs (1905), who stated that the double inoculation method can be complicated by T. theileri; Rao & Ayyar (1931) who stated that T. theileri parasitaemias occur during virus production; and Uganda (1932) where a cow inoculated with viraemic blood had a "violent" attack of rinderpest associated with a high parasitaemia.

Episodes in Tanzania associated with the "double inoculation" method of vaccination against rinderpest were investigated more thoroughly than elsewhere (Hornby & Bailey 1929; Hornby 1930, 1936, 1949; Hornby et al. 1934). Cattle in which these unusual reactions were likely to occur were noted to have originated from one particular district. Believing that these animals were not infected with T. theileri and that concurrent primary infection with both T. theileri and rinderpest virus was a fatal combination, action was taken to avoid this circumstance. Cattle were therefore either given an inoculation of known parasitaemic blood some days before the virus inoculation, or the virus was passed through goats to eliminate the trypanosome, or the viraemic bovine blood was swabbed onto nasal mucous membrane instead of being injected. As a result the second temperature rise associated with T. theileri-like trypanosomes ceased to occur.

As transmission of T. theileri-like trypanosomes alone to presumed susceptible cattle has never provoked more than a febrile reaction (e.g. Behn 1912) and high parasitaemias have been reported without noticeable associated symptoms (e.g. Ewing & Carnahan 1967), a likelihood exists that the destruction of lymphocytes by rinderpest virus (Refik Bey 1902) has an immunosuppressant effect. The same phenomenon may be responsible for the other allegations of pathogenicity of these trypanosomes. From the evidence available, therefore, T. theileri-like trypanosomes may be considered normally non-pathogenic, excepting in circumstances of development forms causing mechanical injury in the brain of the host.

IMMUNOLGY

The only immunological studies available appear to be the few miscellaneous references relating to serological diagnosis. Gray & Nixon (1967) failed to detect infections in calves born to infected dams and therefore considered prenatal infections unlikely. Since calves, however, could be naturally infected as early as one month of age, it seemed also likely that no immunity was acquired from the dams.

Once infected, an animal can remain demonstrably so on culture for periods of at least one year (Vrijburg 1912), two years (Saisawa et al. 1933; Gray & Nixon 1967), three years (Wells 1971b), six years (Robinson 1923) or for life (Carpano 1913). Allegations that infected cattle may cease to be parasitaemic after a period of time, e.g. Vrijburg (1912), may be based on an incomplete knowledge of natural variations in level of parasitaemia. There is therefore no evidence that a sterile immunity may occur, and T. theileri-like trypanosomes appear well adapted to their hosts.

EPIDEMIOLOGY

1. Geographical incidence

Most of the evidence of geographical distribution (see appropriate section) does not indicate the incidence. Not only do the methods of blood examination and culture vary, but the ages of the animals sampled and the season of the year may not be recorded, when both may also affect the numbers of animals found infected. Sufficient cultural evidence exists, however, to show that in the same geographical area the incidence of infection in adult cattle may vary from 100% to a level not detected on one or more examinations. Reid et al. (1966), for example, used a culture technique to sample four groups of adult cattle in East Africa within a three-month period. The numbers of animals found infected were, respectively, 34 out of 35, 12 out of 30, 5 out of 30, and nil out of 33. The last herd result was later confirmed on a second occasion.

2. Age incidence

The highest incidence of infection in a herd of cattle appears to occur in adult animals. Indication of this has been given by Knuth (1910), Crawley (1912a, b), Johns (1913) and Glaser (1922). More specifically, Reid et al. (1966, 1970) in East Africa found that the youngest calf infected in a herd was two and a half months old, thereafter there was a gradual increase in the incidence with age, 34 of 35 cattle over two years of age being infected. Gray & Nixon (1967), in Nigeria, found 35 of 47 cattle infected over one year of age, and 7 of 20 cattle of less than one year.

Wells et al. (1970) in Colombia studied 28 animals in one herd and 30 in another. In both herds all animals older than 30 months were found infected (all of 17 and all of 7), while of animals younger than 30 months, 4 of 11 and 11 of 23 were found infected, respectively. Infections have however been found in foetuses (e.g. Lundholm et al. 1959) or in new-born calves (e.g. Anon. 1966; Lamy & Bouley 1967).

3. Levels of parasitaemia

Some quantitative information was obtained by Johns (1913), who found a variation of between 2 and 21 trypanosomes in each 10 ml of whole blood, using his centrifugal technique. Several authors have determined the minimum infective dose of blood to culture, from which a level of parasitaemia can be inferred, e.g. Richardson (1930, 1948), but Wells (1971b) carried out infectivity titrations on the blood of an infected cow in Scotland using series of blood agar cultures and concluded that in the months of examination (July and August) the maximum parasitaemia exhibited on any one of a total of 27 days was one infective trypanosome per ml of peripheral blood. The level of parasitaemia can, however, vary seasonally in temperate climates. Behn (1910a), Knuth (1910), Robinson (1923), Saisawa et al. (1933), Schmid (1938), Julian (1971) and particularly Crawley (1912a, b) commented that the trypanosomes appeared more difficult to demonstrate on culture in winter. Wells (1971b) followed the parasitaemia of a single infected cow in Scotland over two and a half years and found the highest parasitaemias in the summer between the months of April and September. Supporting evidence was obtained from a further seven cattle (see also section: culture). In tropical areas, however, seasons may be mainly characterized by rainfall and less by variation of temperature. Gray & Nixon (1967), in Nigeria, detected no regular seasonal variation on culture of cattle blood, but Curasson (1925) in West Africa and Keymer (1969) in Central Africa both found trypanosomes more easy to find on blood smears in the rainy seasons.

4. The effect of chemotherapeutic agents

There is no evidence that trypanocidal drugs currently or formerly used for the control of salivarian trypanosomes have any great effect on T. theileri-like parasitaemias in cattle. Vrijburg (1912) treated two calves with trypan blue, but obtained cultures successfully one week later. Hornby et al. (1934) took blood from a cow infected with T. congolense, T. vivax and T. theileri-like trypanosomes and stored it for one hour after adding tartar emetic. Only T. theileri-like trypanosomes survived. The same trypanosomes have probably been commonly noted during field trials of new trypanocidal drugs, but have not attracted comment. They were seen in Nigeria, for example, during a trial of a suramin-metamidium complex (Ferguson - personal communication). Lastly, Onyango (1967) found that diminazene aceturate had an "insignificant" effect on T. theileri-like infections of six cattle at a dosage rate of 7.0 mg/kg, although T. congolense group infections were eliminated in the same animals. Success has only been claimed with "novarsenol" (an arsenical not listed in the British Veterinary Codex), which has never been used as a trypanocide in the field. Sergent et al. (1945) eliminated a T. theileri-like infection in a calf with this drug on the basis of evidence of subsequent absence of a patent parasitaemia and loss of infectivity of peripheral blood to another calf.

Splitter & Soulsby (1967) examined the effect of antibiotics on culture forms. Penicillin, dihydrostreptomycin, oxytetracycline and chloramphenicol failed to have an effect at the concentrations used, but nystatin was found to be lethal to the T. theileri-like trypanosomes under examination at 200 units/ml or higher, and lower concentration resulted in suppression of multiplication. Van Der Maaten & Malmquist (1969) were concerned with the elimination of these trypanosomes as contaminants of cell cultures. They found amphotericin B a more active trypanocidal drug than nystatin when used at concentrations which were not inhibitory to their embryonic spleen and bovine kidney cell cultures.

5. Natural transmission

The vectors of T. theileri-like trypanosomes are commonly accepted to be horse-flies (Diptera: Tabanidae). The opinion is based principally on the work of Nöller (1925), who used three cultures derived from wild Haematopota pluvialis caught near Berlin to attempt infection of four calves. Wallace (1962) examined this evidence and concluded "the fact of transmission of Trypanosoma theileri from tabanid flies to cattle appears to be proved", but qualified this by saying "the identity of the insect stage, however, is not so clear". The evidence for the means of natural transmission of T. theileri-like trypanosomes merits further examination.

Arthropod species of different families may act as vectors for apparently similar trypanosome species. Baker (1956), for example, found that T. avium was transmitted in Hertfordshire, England, by a hippoboscid Ornithomyia avicularia, while in Canada Bennett (1961) considered that hippoboscids were not usually involved in his study location, but found consistent development of avian trypanosomes in several species of ornithophilic simuliids. An assumption of arthropod host family or species specificity even in a single location may be unjustified. T. cruzi has the capability of infecting more than one species of triatomid bug (Hemiptera: Reduviidae), and at least experimental transmissions of T. cruzi-like organisms have been achieved between animal and animal using hard ticks (Acari: Ixodidae) (Pifano 1941) which can theoretically be found in the same localities. In relation to T. theileri-like trypanosomes, few field observations exist of the distribution and availability of possible vectors in relation to infected animals.

The evidence for the natural transmission of T. theileri-like trypanosomes may therefore be summarized as follows:

Transmission by arthropods

(i) Louse flies (Diptera: Hippoboscidae). Theiler (1903, 1909) considered that he had proven Hippobosca rufipes and H. maculata to be transmitters of Trypanosoma theileri (see also Laveran 1903). His experimental animals, however, could have been infected prior to the experiment and, if he was successful, it could only have been through "mechanical" as opposed to cyclical transmission. Lühs (1905), Knuth (1910) and Kearney (1926) all considered hippoboscids to be likely vectors, but Van Saceghem (1922) in Rwanda and Nöller (1925) in Germany stated that a high incidence of T. theileri-like infections in cattle were possible in areas where hippoboscids were rare or absent. Baker (1956) considered that the possibility of a hippoboscid transmitting T. theileri was worth re-examination. Keymer (1969), however, examined 132 Echestypus paradoxus which had fed on duikers (Sylvicarpa grimmia) infected with T. theileri-like trypanosomes and failed to find any trypanosomatid infections.

(ii) Muscid flies (Diptera: Muscidae). Behn (1911) thought Stomoxys calcitrans a likely vector, and Jegen (1924) demonstrated an incidence of trypanosomatid parasites in this species both of choanomastigote and epimastigote form. Glaser (1922) examined 85 Haematobia serrata collected from stables housing infected cattle and found no flagellates. After feeding ten of the same species on "vigorous" cultures of T. theileri-like trypanosomes there was a survival of the flagellates in the alimentary canal for up to 48 hours. The same author also examined 92 Musca domestica, but only found frequent Herpetomonas muscae domesticae infections. Buxton (1955) considered that there was no evidence of Glossina spp. (tsetse) transmitting members of the subgenus Megatrypanum, but noted that "under natural conditions tsetse flies of several species must from time to time ingest a variety of other trypanosomes" (i. e. other than T. grayi and salivarian trypanosomes) e. g. "T. theileri".

(iii) Horse-flies (Diptera: Tabanidae). Knuth & Rauchbaar (1910a) found a trypanosomatid infection of Haematopota pluvialis and suggested that it was the insect stage of T. theileri.

Nöller (1916) described flagellate "resting stages", which he considered to be metacyclic forms of T. theileri, in the hind gut of Tabanus glaucopis. He cultured these forms on blood agar plates at room temperature and believed his cultures to be morphologically identical to those obtained from culturing parasitaemic cattle blood. Later (1925) he examined "numerous" Haematopota pluvialis in the neighbourhood of Berlin and found four infected with flagellates. From three of these, each obtained from a different area, he isolated trypanosomatids on blood agar plates, again finding them morphologically similar to cultures of flagellates derived from the peripheral blood of cattle. Plate washings pooled from these three strains were then used to inoculate calves which were assumed to be free of infection (see section:

prenatal transmission). Cultures from plates kept at room temperatures appeared to infect a 5-day-old calf, but failed to infect a 13-day-old animal. A further 5-day-old calf appeared to be successfully infected from plates which had been kept at 32°C in order to use cultures containing a greater proportion of trypomastigote forms. A bullock 7 - 9 months old was unsuccessfully inoculated twice at an interval of one month, but a third inoculatiion after a further interval of a month appeared successful. This inoculum had been obtained from a plate originating from only one of the Haematopota strains. This culture was 31 days old on the passage used and showed rounded-off, barley-corn-shaped flagellates which "abundantly resembled the resting forms of the flagellates in the gut of the gad-fly". These forms either had the kinetoplast at the posterior end or just anterior to the nucleus. Nöller had not noticed them in the other inocula used in his experiments, but these had been derived from cultures not more than 10 days old in passages used.

Jegen (1924) found flagellates in 14 out of 60 Haematopota pluvialis, but was unable to decide whether they were parasites of the fly alone. He noted a similarity to T. gravi infections in tsetse fly.

In Java (Djawa) Nieschulz (1931) found flagellates in Tabanus rubidus, T. striatus and T. rufiventris, which he considered to be associated with Trypanosoma theileri. Kraneveld (1931) also suspected tabanids to be the transmitters following the detection on culture of a "high" incidence of T. theileri-like trypanosomes in the cattle and buffalo populations of Java. On preliminary investigations he found 636 Tabanus striatus out of 3504 dissected to have trypanosomatid infections and likewise 1048 out of 4862 Tabanus rubidus. The flagellates from both tabanid species were cultured on blood agar, and Kraneveld stated that their appearance resembled T. theileri-like organisms cultured from the peripheral blood of cattle. Kraneveld found a smaller incidence of flagellates of the same appearance in Tabanus rufiventris, T. brunnipennis, T. basalis and Haematopota javana, but less numbers were examined of these species. He then attempted transmission experiments using large numbers of wild Tabanus striatus which he allowed to feed daily on the shaven skin of two buffaloes and an ox. Two of the three animals appeared to have been infected by this means, but as care had been taken to prevent insect faeces from contaminating the skin of the host there was also the appearance that infection had been caused by inoculative transmission. He also demonstrated the ability of flagellates in the intestinal contents of Tabanus striatus to penetrate the mucous membranes of the mouth and infect an ox and a water buffalo. Similarly, another water buffalo was infected by the flagellates penetrating the mucous membrane of the vagina. No infections resulted from subcutaneous inoculations.

Similar experiments with Tabanus rubidus had no success, and Kraneveld could only conclude that the flagellates parasitizing this species were not vector stages of bovine trypanosomes.

Kraneveld admitted that he was unable to distinguish between trypanosomatids which were parasites of flies themselves and those which were developmental forms of T. theileri-like trypanosomes. In flies which had been used successfully to transmit trypanosomes he saw, in particular, large, slow-moving, epimastigote forms, very mobile, small forms, and rounded off forms with flagella. The first two types were in both mid and hind guts, while the third was found with the first two in the insect faeces.

Packchanian (1957) examined trypanosomatid parasites of Tabanus atratus in the U. S. A., and considered that the flagellates seen both in the initial smear of the insect gut and in subsequent cultures were "indistinguishable from the cultural form of Trypanosoma theileri isolated from cows" which the author had examined several years previously. Page (in press) had a similar experience culturing flagellates from the hind gut of Lepiselaga crassipes on the Atlantic coast of Colombia.

Clarkson (1966 - personal communication) attempted to infect wild populations of Haematopota pluvialis with T. theileri-like organisms. Even though his experimentation was only exploratory in nature and there was no clear result, he showed that feeding flies on parasitaemic defibrinated blood, kept at 37° C, through membranes was a possible technique.

(iv) Other Diptera. Mayer (1912) alone has suggested mosquitoes as vectors. Kraneveld (1931) suggested simuliids in addition to tabanids because of their habit of feeding on eye secretions and also because experimentally he had shown that penetration of mucous membranes by T. theileri-like trypanosomes was possible.

(v) Ticks (Acari: Ixodidae). O'Farrell (1913) described Crithidia hyalommae as strictly a parasitic flagellate of Hyalomma aegyptium, occurring in haemocoelic fluid, salivary glands, ovary, oviducts and ova of the host. Carpano (1932) saw a similar flagellate in one of 20 ticks of the same species in Libya, and offered the theory that it was the vector of T. theileri. Reichenow (1940), however, discounted this, believing that if T. theileri and C. hyallomae were identical, then the infection was accidental. Parasites of the genus Blastocrithidia have, however, been reported in other ticks, e. g. B. christophersi in Rhipicephalus sanguineus and B. haemaphysalidis in Haemaphysalis flava (Wallace 1966). Whether they represent the vector forms of trypanosomes infecting the host of the tick species is unknown.

Prenatal transmission

The detection of infections in bovine foetuses or new-born calves with T. theileri-like trypanosomes has been reported. Dikmans et al. (1957) found such flagellates in a foetal stomach, Lundholm et al. (1959) found them contaminating primary monolayers of foetal bovine kidney cells; in Virginia (Anon. 1966) patent parasitaemias were found in six new-born calves, and Lamy & Bouley (1967) found a heavy parasitaemia in one new-born calf. The preponderance of evidence, however, indicates that prenatal infection is an abnormal method of transmission (e.g. see Reid et al. 1966; Gray & Nixon 1967; Wells, Lumsden & MacNeillage 1968).

6. Artificial transmission

T. theileri-like trypanosomes appear to have been successfully transmitted to experimental bovine animals by means of whole parasitaemic blood, cultures of trypanosomes from peripheral blood maintained at 32° C or 37° C, cultures of trypanosomes obtained from peripheral blood of cattle, cultures from intestinal contents of Tabanidae and maintained at room temperature, and the intestinal content of tabanid flies. Comparison of results is often difficult owing to incomplete records of experimental methods, but a possible consistent failure has been the inadequate examination of animals for trypanosome infections before the start of experimentation, although calves seem mainly to have been chosen to minimize this possibility.

(i) Transmission using whole parasitaemic blood. The detection of a patent parasitaemia may have been assisted in some experiments by the concurrent inoculation of a pathogen, e.g. rinderpest virus (Schein 1907; Curasson 1925) or babesia (Dios & Zuccarini 1924). Carpano (1924) even gave the opinion that the detection of a patent parasitaemia depended on this happening and even then did not reliably occur. Several authors, however, have recorded no difficulty in infecting either entire or splenectomized cattle with whole parasitaemic blood and detecting infection on blood smears, e.g. Theiler (1903), Behn (1912), Bonger (1913), Van Saceghem (1922), Levine et al. (1956), Iwata et al. (1959), and Hoyte (1968 - personal communication). Others did not succeed in all cases e.g. Behn (1910c), Teague & Clark (1918), Hornby et al. (1934) and Keymer (1969), while Holmes (1904) failed with each of four animals.

Keymer's attempts (1969) were of additional interest, because he was attempting transmission from a duiker to a calf. He himself, however, doubted his one apparently successful result, as the calf first showed a large form, of 80 μ body length, only four and a half days after injection of parasitaemic blood. As he considered that these forms represented long standing infections, he felt that the experimental animal might have been previously infected.

The alleged failure to transmit the trypanosome might have been proved successful if culture diagnosis had been used. Vrijburg (1912) and Wells (1969) only succeeded in demonstrating transmission to calves by cultural methods.

(ii) Transmission using cultures maintained at 32° C and 37° C. Nöller (1925) cultured flagellates from wild Haematopota pluvialis (see section: epidemiology - natural transmission - horse-flies), maintaining blood agar plates at 32° C before preparing an inoculum and infecting a calf.

Hulliger (1964 - personal communication) infected a calf but with T. theileri-like trypanosomes, which had appeared as contaminants on a leucocyte monolayer kept at 37°C. Splitter & Soulsby (1967) used their "large volume" culture at 37°C (see section: culture) to infect a calf in which immunological competence had been temporarily impaired by irradiation from two cobalt-60 sources. Cross et al. (1968) used one of Splitter's media containing trypanosomes to infect one splenectomized calf, and infected another with buffy coat culture fluids which contained trypanosomes.

(iii) Transmission using cultures maintained at room temperatures. Miyajima (1907) detected patent parasitaemias in two calves out of three after inoculating them with broth cultures consisting of motile trypanosomes "in abundance". Martini (1909) successfully infected calves using a broth culture maintained at 29-31°C, but at these temperatures he might have begun to influence the number of trypomastigote forms present. Kohl-Yakimoff, Yakimoff & Bekensky (1913a) also claimed to have infected a calf, using a broth culture, but gave no experimental details. Nöller (1925) cultured flagellates from three Haematopota pluvialis onto blood agar plates, and from growths obtained at room temperature infected one calf out of two at the first attempt, and appeared to infect an older bullock at the third attempt (see section: epidemiology - natural transmission-horse-flies).

Both Behn (1912) and Vrijburg (1912) failed to infect calves with cultures maintained at room temperature, although both authors had been successful with whole parasitaemic blood. Likewise, an annual report (India 1940) recorded that "no infection could be produced by the inoculation of healthy bulls with the crithidial (i.e. epimastigote) forms".

(iv) Transmission using intestinal contents of tabanid flies. The successful experiments of Kraneveld (1931) using intestinal contents of Tabanus striatus have already been described (section epidemiology - natural transmission - horse-flies).

STORAGE OF STRAINS

Study of T. theileri-like trypanosomes most easily commences from isolation of the forms in peripheral blood. The survival of these trypanosomes in whole blood at different temperatures is important, particularly in the field, to determine maximum permissible time lag between collection and inoculation of cultures without loss of infectivity. After isolating T. theileri-like trypanosomes, investigators have maintained them by continuous subculture at approximately weekly intervals, e.g. Crawley (1912a, b) and Nöller (1925), or even for a period of years (Herbert 1965a). There appear to be only two references to storage at low temperatures (Splitter & Soulsby 1967; Wells 1971a).

T. theileri-like trypanosomes have been seen to retain motility in wet preparations of peripheral blood for at least one hour by Teague &

Clark (1918), for "some hours" by Schein (1907), and 18 - 36 hours under a cemented cover-slip (Carpano 1913). Several authors have commented on the retention of infectivity to culture of peripheral blood after storage at different temperatures. For example, at temperatures approximating 4° C, blood retained some infectivity for culture media for a maximum of 4 days (Crawley 1912), 5 days (Saisawa et al. 1933), 7 days (Theiler 1903), 21 days (Woo et al. 1970) or 27 days (Vrijburg 1912). At room temperature, findings have also been widely divergent, e.g. 6 hours (Leach 1964), 24 - 30 hours (Johns 1913), 3 days (Crawley 1912; Saisawa et al. 1933), 7 days (Theiler 1903), and over three weeks (Vrijburg 1912). At 37° C Crawley (1912) and Saisawa et al. (1933) agree on a maximum of 24 hours, but Vrijburg (1912) gave 4 days.

For low temperature storage of isolates, Splitter & Soulsby (1967) stored cultures by mixing them with glycerine, phosphate buffered glucose and saline (pH 7.5), and cooling the mixture to -20° C in a commercial deep-freeze without regard to speed of cooling. The trypanosomes were then taken rapidly to -70° C in solid CO_2 and ethanol. "Motility and ability to grow in culture were unaffected by storage at -20° C for 24 hours. Storage at -20° C for 7 and 14 days markedly reduced motility, and cultures of such material were negative. After 30 days storage at -20° C, organisms were no longer viable and they failed to grow in cultures". Cultures which had been quickly frozen to -70° C were readily subcultured after at least 50 days storage at this temperature. Wells (1971a) used the method of storage in dry ice (-79° C) described by Cunningham et al. (1963). Differences were that he froze the liquid of blood agar cultures in place of peripheral blood, dimethylsulphoxide replaced glycerol as the cryoprotectant in 125 of 135 frozen populations, and of the remaining ten, four were stored in liquid N_2 (-196° C). They were found to retain infectivity up to four and a half years. Some loss of infectivity was noticed in 15 stabilates, but there was no relationship between these and the method of storage or their age.

LIFE CYCLE

Carpano (1932) postulated a series of events from his own observations in the brain and lymph nodes of cattle and of trypanosomatid infections in Hyalomma aegyptium. Reichenow (1940) discounted both the idea of multiplication in fixed tissues and of tick transmission, but Hoare (1936) accepted a conclusion by Carpano that T. theileri behaved similarly to Trypanosome cruzi in the mammalian host. The information relevant to the life cycle of T. theileri-like organisms may be summarized and discussed as follows:

1. Stages in fixed tissues

As the parasitaemia in the mammalian host is normally only detectable on culture, and forms in division are seen only exceptionally in the peripheral blood, multiplication of the trypanosomes in fixed tissues can be argued to be analogous to species in the stercorarian subgenera Herpetomonas, e.g. T. nabiasi (Molyneux 1969), and Schizotrypanum, e.g. T. cruzi (Chagas 1909). Some support is given by the two descriptions of T. theileri-like organisms in lymph nodes (Carpano 1932; Gallo 1938). The conglomerations described in brain tissue could be considered accidental and possibly analogous to reports of Theileri schizonts (e.g. Carmichael 1939) or collections of erythrocytes infected with Babesia spp. (e.g. Zlotnick 1953).

Descriptions of dividing forms in the peripheral blood have mostly been from high parasitaemias associated with concurrent infections of rinderpest virus. Either this is an exaggeration of the same events at sub-patent parasitaemias, or developmental stages normally occurring in fixed tissues are being revealed. The latter is assumed in the present account. Lühs (1905) believed that division could either be longitudinal, giving epimastigote daughters of equal size, or transverse, giving epimastigote daughters of unequal size. Reichenow (1940) examined slides supplied by Hornby, and described unequal division only. He theorized that, of the two epimastigote daughters, the larger eventually became the giant trypomastigote forms of chronic infections, while the smaller were capable of further division. Comparison of the drawings of unequal division made by both Lühs and Reichenow shows remarkable similarity (fig. 2). The process could follow on the events in fixed tissues described by Carpano (1932) involving amastigote forms.

2. Forms in peripheral blood

The morphology of the organisms most usually described in the peripheral blood follows from Reichenow's theory, including the description of epimastigote forms. The quantitative and qualitative differences of cultures from peripheral blood of an infected animal reported by Crawley (1909) and Wells (1971a, b) (see section: culture) can be expected to relate to the morphology of peripheral blood forms, and their presence or absence may account for the irregularities seen in transmission experiments from bovine animal to bovine animal using whole blood. From this point of view, the two morphologically different populations of trypanosomes described by Woo et al. (1970) in the blood of five cows can be argued as more likely to be stages in the life-cycle of the same trypanosome rather than representing two different species.

3. Transmission from mammalian host to a vector

Wells (1971b) theorized that his cultures obtained during late summer in Scotland with the capability of long survival were derived from peripheral blood forms infective to a vector. The vector can be anticipated to be infected from a blood meal from an infected host.

4. Forms in an insect vector

The culture of trypanosomes at room temperature is considered to be analogous to multiplication in the insect vector (Wenyon 1926), but whereas the morphogenesis in culture described first by Crawley (1912) and later by Herbert (1965a) rationalizes the majority of observations, no indication was made by these authors that the metacyclic stage was reached.

Nöller (1925) discusses the possibility of metacyclic forms occurring in cultures at room temperature. He believed that the "barley corn" forms in a 31-day-old culture (Nöller 1925) were equivalent to the forms that he had seen lining the hind gut of tabanids and from which he had made cultures. The forms described by Nöller could also be the same as the "rounded off" or oval, flagellated forms seen, for example, by Kraneveld (1931) in the hind gut of Tabanus striatus, by Patton (1909) in the hind gut of Tabanus hilarius and an unidentified Tabanus sp., and by Bruce et al. (1911) in Tabanus secedens. Wells (1971b) found that his blood agar cultures obtained in late summer with the capability of surviving long periods of time also developed forms fitting Nöller's description of "barley corn". In such "old" cultures he also commonly found populations of small, very active flagellates, as described on a single occasion from a 47-day-old blood agar plate by Nöller (1917). These could conceivably be equivalent to the active flagellates seen in the mid gut of Tabanus striatus by Kraneveld (1931).

Support for the hypothesis of Nöller's barley corn" forms being the metacyclic stage of T. theileri-like trypanosomes can be gained by consideration of the metacyclic stage of other trypanosomes, the development of which occurs in the hind gut of insect vectors, and where knowledge concurrently exists of the appearance of the same forms in culture media, e.g. T. avium (Baker 1956, 1966), T. conorhini (Deane & Kirchner 1963), T. cruzi (Camago 1964), T. danilewskyi (Thomson 1908; quoted by Hoare 1923), T. grayi (Hoare 1923), and T. zapi (Davis 1952). In all cases metacyclic forms occurred in primary culture, and, despite differences of fixing and staining, the metacyclic forms described for T. avium, T. lewisi and T. melophagium in particular have resemblance to the "barley corn" forms described by Nöller.

Wallace (1962), however, believed that these "barley corn" forms must have been choanomastigote in form, representing a tryposomatid species of the genus Crithidia. Certainly, Nöller did not eliminate the possibility that his cultures were of more than one species. Thomson (1933), for example, clearly figured choanomastigote forms in a tabanid (T. africanus), as did Wallace himself in T. epistates. Wallace described the possibility that a "cryptic" infection of T. theileri-like trypanosome forms in the hind gut of the vector may have in its turn overwhelmed the choanomastigote forms in the culture. In balance it appears likely that Wallace was mistaken in his surmise of the nature of Nöller's "resting forms", but final resolution of this point will depend on the further work on trypanosomatid infections of tabanids which Wallace himself strongly advocated.

The significance of the thickening at the tip of the flagellum of T. theileri-like trypanosomes occasionally reported has not been discussed by any worker. Similar phenomena described for Crithidia fasciculata by Kusel et al. (1967) and for T. lewisi by Molyneux (1968, 1969) were interpreted by the latter author as an adaptation of the parasite to life in the vector, assisting attachment to the wall of the hind gut.

5. Transmission from a vector to a susceptible host

The evidence suggests that several species of the family Tabanidae are vectors of T. theileri-like trypanosomes. An obstacle to further work is the present failure to develop laboratory colonies of any member of this family. In addition, no studies exist of the habits of tabanids in relation to their hosts; these would obviously affect the sites of deposition of metacyclic forms in insect faeces. Assumption has to be made that this occurs in sites where the host may lick, following the observation by Kraneveld (1931) that an animal was apparently infected by placing intestinal contents of Tabanus striatus in contact with mucous membrane of the mouth, or by penetration of broken skin.

CONCLUSIONS

Knowledge of the biology of these large trypanosomes of cattle is inadequate to determine whether the phenomena relate to a single trypanosome species or to a group of similar organisms. The study of DNA components may, however, be informative. The use of the term "T. theileri-like", first suggested by Keymer (1967), is therefore justified, reserving the species name Trypanosoma theileri for Theiler's observations in South Africa. This decision requires a re-appraisal of the taxonomy of the subgenus Megatrypanum.

T. theileri-like trypanosomes present problems approachable from three main viewpoints: first, an approach seeking knowledge of the biological characteristics of the T. theileri-like trypanosomes and their affinities to trypanosome species found elsewhere in the animal kingdom; secondly, resolution of the question of the possibility of interference from members of the subgenus with the serological diagnosis of salivarian trypanosomes; thirdly, T. theileri-like trypanosomes as a training ground for workers in temperate countries wishing to work on applied problems of trypanosomal diseases in the tropics. Any of these approaches is certain to be rewarding.

Table 1

Records of T. theileri-like trypanosomes observed by direct microscopy in the peripheral blood of artiodactyls other than domestic oxen (Bos taurus and Bos indicus), using the nomenclature of Morris (1965) for mammalian hosts.

FAMILY	HOST SPECIES	TRYPANOSOME	REFERENCE
Suidae (8 species)	-	-	-
Tayassuidae (2 species)	-	-	-
Hippopotanidae	-	-	-
Camelidae (6 species)	Camelus dromedarius (Arabian camel)	T. theileri	Roetti (1940)
Tragulidae (4 species)	Tragulus javanicus (Lesser Malay chevrotain)	T. ingens	Dodd (1912)
Cervidae (41 species)	Mazama rufa toba* (Brocket deer)	T. mazamarum**	Mazza et al. (1932)
	Mazama nevorivagus*	T. mazamarum	Mazza et al. (1932)
	Mazama simplicornis* (Brocket deer)	T. mazamarum	Deane (1961)
		'theileri-like'	Deane (1967)
Giraffidae (2 species)	-	-	-
Antilocapridae (1 specie)	-	-	-
Bovidae (128 species)	Tragelaphus spekei (Sitatunga)	T. ingens	Duke (1912) Kinghorn & Yorke (1929)
		T. tragelaphi	Kinghorn et al. (1913) Hoare (1929)

Table 1 cont.

FAMILY	HOST SPECIES	TRYPANOSOME	REFERENCE	
	Tragelaphus scriptus (Bushbuck)	T. theileri	Dutton et al.	(1906)
			Dutton et al.	(1907)
			Baker	(1958)
		T. ingens	Bruce et al.	(1909b)
			Fraser & Duke	(1912)
			Old	(1915)
			Hoare	(1929)
		T. tragelaphi	Hoare	(1929)
			Morris	(1932)
			Neitz	(1933)
	Tragelaphus strepsiceros (Greater Kudu)	T. theileri	Travassos Santos Dias	(1960)
	Tragelaphus oryx (Eland)	T. ingens	Old	(1915)
	Tragelaphus sp.	T. tragelaphus	Schwetz	(1931)
	Bubalus bubalis (Asiatic buffalo)	T. theileri	Pease	(1909)
			Haughwout & Youngberg	(1920)
			Kraneveld	(1931)
	Syncerus caffer (African buffalo)	T. theileri	Baker	(1958)
	Bison bonasus (European bison)	T. wrublewskii	Wrublewski	(1912)
	Cephalophus dorsalis (Bay duiker)	T. ingens	Rodhain	(1916)

Table 1 cont.

FAMILY	HOST SPECIES	TRYPANOSOME	REFERENCE	
	Sylvicapra grimmia (Grey duiker)	T. theileri	Rodhain et al.	(1913);
			Travassos Santos Dias	(1960)
		T. ingens	Rodhain et al.	(1912, 1913)
			Bruce et al.	(1913)
			Travassos Santos Dias	(1960)
		T. tragelaphi	Travassos Santos Dias	(1960)
		T. cephalophi	Bruce et al.	(1913);
			Travassos Santos Dias	(1960)
		'theileri-like'	Keymer	(1969)xxx
	Kobus ellipsiprymnus (Waterbuck)	T. theileri	Thomas & Neitz	(1933)
		T. ingens	Bruce et al.	(1914)
	Kobus kob (Kob)	T. theileri	Baker	(1958);
			Uganda	(1961)
		T. tragelaphi	Morris	(1932);
			Morriss	(1940)//
			Brocklesby & Vidler	(1965)
	Kobus vardoni (Puku)	"large trypanosomes"	Rodhain et al.	(1913)
		"theileri-like"	Keymer	(1969)
		T. ingens	Neveu-Lemaire	(1943)/

Table 1 cont.

FAMILY	HOST SPECIES	TRYPANOSOME	REFERENCE	
	Redunca arundinum (Reedbuck)	T. theileri	Kleine & Fischer	(1912)
		T. ingens	Bruce et al.	(1909b, 1919)
	Redunca sp.	T. tragelaphi	Morriss	(1940) ††
	Hippotragus equinus (Roan antelope)	T. theileri	Neveu-Lemaire	(1943) †
	Ourebia curebi (Oribi)	T. ingens	Neveu-Lemaire	(1943) †
	Ourebia sp.	T. ingens	Bruce et al.	(1913)
	Raphicerus campestris (Steinbok)	T. theileri	Schwetz	(1931)
	Nesotragus moschatus (Suni)	T. theileri	Travassos Santos Dias	(1960)
		T. ingens	Travassos Santos Dias	(1960)
		T. cephalophi	Travassos Santos Dias	(1960)

* species not recognized by Morris (1965).

** also spelt 'mazamorum' in the same article.

*** Keymer (1969) saw forms resembling T. theileri, ingens, tragelaphi and cephalophi commonly and referred to them as 'theileri-like'. See text.

† Neveu-Lemaire (1943) included these isolations in an appendix to his textbook, additional to those listed elsewhere in this table. He does not, however, state the source of his information.

†† Morris (1932) and Morriss (1940) are probably the same person. The second reference is a personal communication to Curasson (1943); his name may be mis-spelt, as both refer to the former Gold Coast.

Table 2

Records of T. theileri-like trypanosomes cultured from the peripheral blood of artiodactyls other than domestic oxen (Bos taurus and Bos indicus)

FAMILY	HOST SPECIES	TRYPANOSOME	REFERENCE	
Cervidae			d'Alessandro (1967-personal communication	
Bovidae	Tragelaphus spekei (Sitatunga)	'theileri-like'	Reid et al.	(1966)
	Tragelaphus scriptus (Bushbuck)	'theileri-like'	Reid et al.	(1966, 1970)
	Bubalus bubalis (Asiatic buffalo)	T. theileri	Kraneveld	(1931)
	* (duiker)	T. cephalophi	Bruce et al.	(1915)
	Sylvicapra grimmia (Grey duiker)	'theileri-like'	Keymer	(1969)

* called Cephalophus grimmi by Bruce but probably Sylvicapra grimmia (see Morris 1965).

<u>Appendix</u>

Published and unpublished records of the demonstration of T. theileri-like trypanosomes in bovine tissues either by direct microscopy or by culture.

The following list is not exhaustive, particularly as there are many unpublished observations, but the cosmopolitan distribution of T. theileri-like trypanosomes is illustrated. The geographical arrangement may also be of use for purposes of reference.

EUROPE

England	Stockman	1910
	Coles	1913
	Joyner	1964 *
	Pierce	1964 *
	Hoyte	1968 *
	Wells et al.	1968
Scotland	Wells et al.	1965, 1968
Northern Ireland	Kerr	1942
	Kerr & Robertson	1943
Eire	Herbert	1961
Denmark	Anon.	1919 **
	Christiansen	1911
Finland	Weber	1909
France	Delanoe	1911
	Galliard	1925
	Lamy & Bouley	1967
Germany	Frank	1909
	Behn	1910, 1912
	Knuth	1910
	Knuth & Rauchbaar	1910
	Knuth et al.	1910

Indonesia cont.		
	Nieschulz	1931
	Kraneveld & Djaenoedin	1932
Japan	Miyajima	1907
	Saisawa et al.	1933
	Sasaki & Nishi	1950
	Iwata et al.	1959
Korea	Yamada Kawamura	1914; 1916
Philippines	Martini	1909
	Haughwout & Youngberg	1920
	Kelser	1927
Singapore	Falshaw & Lingard	1907
U. S. S. R.	Lühs	1905
	Dudukalov	1908
	Dschunkowsky & Lühs	1909
	Wrublewsky	1909
	Dudukalov & Dudulakova	1910
	Sadowsky Marzinowsky	1910; 1911
	Stolnikoff	1911
	Yakimov & Shokhor	1913
	Kohl-Yakimoff, Yakimoff & Bekensky	1913
	Kohl-Yakimoff, Yakimoff & Shokhor	1913
	Yakimoff & Shokhor	1916
	Sassouchin & Matwejeff	1922
	Paratschouk	1924
	Parzwanidze	1925
	Yakimoff & Rastegaieff	1925
	Yakimoff et al.	1925

U. S. S. R. cont.	Belikov	1926
	Dratchinskii & Markov	1927
	Maliavkine	1926
	Yakimov et al.	1926
	Bozrzeff	1928
	Florinsky	1928
	Radkewitsch	1928
	Beresine	1930
	Sudachenkov	1932
	Yakimov et al.	1933
	Sprinholz-Schmidt	1938
Vietnam	Schein	1907

OCEANIC

Australia	Turner & Nurnane	1930 a, b
	Mulhearn (unpublished information quoted by Seddon 1952)	1942

AFRICA

Algeria	Sergent & Sergent	1911
	Sergent et al.	1945
	Vincent	1968 *
Angola	Mendes et al.	1909
Congo Republic	Dutton et al.	1906
	Dutton et al.	1907
	Rodhain et al.	1912, 1913
	Rodhain	1916
	Schwetz	1927, 1928 1930, 1931
Egypt	Carpano	1932
	Egypt	1942
	Ezzart	1961

Ethiopia	Carpano	1913, 1924, 1932
	Caccavella	1939
French Equatorial	Curasson	1925 ≁
	Delpy	1931
French West	Malbrant <u>et al.</u>	1939 ≁
Ghana	Robinson	1929
Kenya	Barnett	1947, 1966*
	Kenya	1957
Lesotho	Neitz	1931, 1933
Malawi	Bruce <u>et al.</u>	1913, 1914, 1915
	Nyasaland, e.g.	1955
	Keymer	1969
Mauritius	Adams	1935
Morocco	F.A.O.	1968
Mozambique	Travassos Santos Dias	1960
Niger	Mornet	1941
Nigeria	Macfie	1913
	Kearney	1926
	Nigeria e.g.	1927
	Glover	1961
	Leach	1964, 1965
	Folkers & Mohammed	1965
	Godfrey <u>et al.</u>	1965
	Wells <u>et al.</u>	1968
	Gray & Nixon	1967
Portugese Guinea	Tendeiro	1945, 1947, 1949
	Ferreira	1948
Rhodesia	Bolton	1965 *
	Keymer	1969

Germany cont.

	Schmitt	1910, 1911
	Nöller	1916, 1917, 1920, 1925
	Trautmann	1922
Greece	Cardamatis & Photinos	1912
Holland	Wester	1911
	Swellengrebel	1911a, b
	Van Der Poel	1912
	Vrijburg	1911, 1912
Iran	F. A. O.	1968
Italy	Carpano	1924
Portugal	Bettencourt & Borge	1912, 1916
Sweden	Anon.	1910
Switzerland	Wyssmann	1935
	Bourgeois	1941
	Stirnimann	1947
	Steck	1966 *

ASIA

China	Heanley	1908
India	Lingard	1903, 1904 1907
	Holmes	1904
	Durrant & Holmes	1904
	Valladares	1909
	Rao & Ayyer	1931
	Naik	1937
	Mahajan	1939
	India	1940
Indonesia	Dodd	1912
	Kraneveld	1931

Rwanda	Van Saceghem	1922
Senegal	Thiroux <u>et al.</u>	1908
	Touré	1968
Somalia	Croverie	1920
	Veri	1920
South Africa	Theiler	1903
	Kehoe	1916
	Robinson	1923
Tanzania	Koch	1904
	Panse	1904
	Stolowsky	1908
	Kleine	1910
	Schoenebeck	1910
	Kleine & Fischer	1912
	Hornby & Bailey	1929
	Hornby <u>et al.</u>	1934
	Reichenow	1940
	Tanganyika, e.g.	1950
Togo	Schilling	1903
Tunisia	Yakimoff & Kohl-Yakimoff	1911a, b
Uganda	Nabarro & Greig	1905
	Bruce <u>et al.</u>	1909b
	Hamerton	1911
	Mackie	1911
	Duke	1912
	Fraser & Duke	1912
	Uganda, e.g.	1925
	Carmichael	1926, 1939
	Hoare	1929
	Richardson	1930, 1948
	Thomson	1931

Uganda cont.	Baker	1958
	Harley	1963
	Reid *et al.*	1966, 1970
Zambia	Montgomery & Kinghorn	1908
	Kinghorn & Yorke	1912
	Kinghorn *et al.*	1913
	Keymer	1969

NORTH AND SOUTH AMERICA

Argentina	Peter	1910
	Dios & Zuccarini	1924
Brazil	Peter	1910
	Carini	1911
Canada	Bowhill	1909a, b
	Watson & Hadwen	1912
	Hall	1953
	Julian	1971
	Woo *et al.*	1970
Colombia	Virviescas	1934
	Wells, Ruiz & Ochoa	1968
	Kuttler *et al.*	1969
	Wells, Betancourt & Page	1970
Guyana	Williams	1971 *
Nicaragua	Gallo	1938
Panama	Teague & Clark	1918
	Panama	1941
Peru	Clarkson & McCabe	1970
Trinidad	Williams	1970 *
Uruguay	Peter	1910

U.S.A.	Crawley	1909, 1912a, b
	Johns	1913, 1914
	Glaser	1922
	Schoening	1925
	Packchanian	1934
	Atchley	1951
	Simpson & Sanders	1951
	Dikmans et al.	1957
	Levine et al.	1956
	Ristic & Trager	1958
	Lundholm et al.	1959
	Simpson & Green	1959
	Benbrook & Sloss	1961
	Anon.	1966
	Ewing & Carnahan	1967
	Splitter et al.	1967
	Cross et al.	1968
	Sollod & Soulsby	1968
Venezuela	Diaz-Ungria et al.	1969

* personal communication.

** personal anonymous communications to Knuth, 1910.

/ the territories named are now independent and the information available is insufficient to state localities in relation to new territorial boundaries.

REFERENCES

Adams, A. R. D. (1935) Trypanosomiasis of stock in Mauritius. II. Observations on the incidence and distribution of trypanosomiasis in cattle. Ann. trop. Med. Parasit. 29, 475-481

Anon. (1966) Trypanosoma theileri in Virginian cattle. Veterinary public health notes. U. S. Department of Health, Education and Welfare; Communicable Disease Centre, February 1966 (also in J. Am. vet. med. Ass. 149, 1294)

Atchley, F. O. (1951) Leucocytozoon andrewsi n. sp., from chickens observed in a survey of blood parasites in domestic animals in South Carolina. J. Parasit. 37, 483-488

Baker, J. R. (1956) Studies on Trypanosoma avium Danilewsky 1885. II. Transmission by Ornithomyia avicularia L. Parasitology 46, 321-334

Baker, J. R. (1958) The examination of blood slides from wild animals. Rep. E. Afr. Trypan. Res. Org., 1956-7 pp. 30-31

Baker, J. R. (1966) Studies on Trypanosoma avium. IV. The development of infective metacyclic trypanosomes in cultures grown in vitro. Parasitology 56, 15-19

Barnett, S. F. (1947) Bovine trypanosomiasis in Kenya with special reference to its treatment with phenanthridinium 897. Vet. Rec. 59, 459-462

Behn, K. (1911) Wachstum von Bluttrypanosomen aus deutschen Rindern auf Blutagar. Berl. tierärztl. Wschr. 27, 307

Behn, P. (1910a) Über Entwicklungsformen des Trypanosoma franki. Berl. tierärztl. Wschr. 26, 809-810

Behn, P. (1910b) Präflagellate Entwicklungsstadien der in deutschen Rindern kuturell nachweisbaren Trypanosomen. Berl. tierärztl. Wschr. 26, 899

Behn, P. (1910c) Infektion eines Kalbes mit Trypanosomen vom Typus des Trypanosoma theileri mittelst Blut von Kühen, in denen nur kulturell Flagellaten nachweisbar waren. Berl. tierärztl. Wschr. 26, 998-1000

Behn, P. (1912) Gehen die bei Rindern kulturell nachweisbaren Flagellaten aus Trypanosomen hervor? Z. Hyg. InfektKrankh. 70, 371-408

Belikov, A. P. (1927) [Distribution of trypanosomiasis in the cattle of the U. S. S. R.] Vestnik Sovrem. Vet. 3, 554-555

Belkewitsch, -. (1915) Quoted by Sprinholz-Schmidt, A. J. (1938)

Benbrook, E. A. & Sloss, M. W. (1961) Veterinary clinical parasitology. 3rd edit. Ames, Iowa: State University Press

Bennett, G. F. (1961) On the specificity and transmission of some avian trypanosomes. Can. J. Zool. 39, 17-33

Berezin, M. I. (1930) [Demonstration of trypanosomes in cattle in the Ural region and studies on their pathogenicity.] Trudy gos. Inst. eksp. Vet. 6, No. 3 pp. 80-84

Bettencourt, A. & Borges, I. (1912) Trypanosomes du sang des bovidés portugais. Bull. Soc. Path. exot. 5, 603-604 & 725
Bettencourt, A. & Borges, I. (1916) Présence de trypanosomes dans le sang des bovidés portugais. Archos R. Inst. bact. Câmara. Pestana 4, 179-181 + 3 plates
Blacklock, R. (1912) The vitality and changes undergone by trypanosomes in the cadaver of the animal host. Ann. trop. Med. Parasit. 8, 55-68
Blanchard, R. (1904) Sur un travail de M. le Dr. Brumpt intitulé: quelques faits relatifs à la transmission de la maladie du sommeil par les mouches tsétsé. Archs Parasit. 8, 573-589
Bonger, C. (1913) Über die Morphologie und das Verhalten der von P. Behn in deutschen Rindern nachgewiesenen Trypanosomen bei künstlicher Infektion. Z. Hyg. InfektKrankh. 75, 101-117
Bourgeois, E. (1941) Zur frage der Pathogenität des Trypanosoma theileri. Schweizer Arch. Tierheilk. 83, 467-469
Bowhill, T. (1909a) Red-water investigations in British Columbia. Health of Animals Report, Canada, 1909
Bowhill, T. (1909b) Note on the occurrence of a large flagellate, associated with a piroplasmata infection in a cow in British Columbia. J. trop. vet. Sci. 4, 104-105
Bozrzeff, -. (1928) Quoted by Sprinholz-Schmid (1938)
Brocklesby, D. W. & Vidler, B. O. (1965) Some parasites of East African wild animals. E. Afr. Wildl. J. 3, 120-122
Bruce, D. (1902) Note on the discovery of a new trypanosoma. Lancet 8th March, 664
Bruce, D., Hamerton, A. E. & Bateman, H. R. (1909a) A trypanosome from Zanzibar. Proc. R. Soc. Ser. B. 81, 14-30
Bruce, D., Hamerton, A. E., Bateman, H. R. & Mackie, F. P. (1909b) Trypanosoma ingens, n. sp. Proc. R. Soc. Ser. B. 81, 323-324
Bruce, D., Hamerton, A. E., Bateman, H. R. & Mackie, F. P. (1910) Trypanosome diseases of domestic animals in Uganda. III. Trypanosoma vivax, Ziemann. Proc. R. Soc. Ser. B. 83, 15-27
Bruce, D., Hamerton, A. E., Bateman, H. R., Mackie, F. P. & Bruce, M. E. (1911) Experiments designed to discover the insect carriers of the trypanosome diseases of domestic animals in Uganda. Rep. sleep. Sickn. Commn. R. Soc. 11, 175-183
Bruce, D., Harvey, D., Hamerton, A. E., Davey, J. B. & Bruce, M. E. (1913) The trypanosomes found in the blood of wild animals living in the sleeping sickness area, Nyasaland. Proc. R. Soc. Ser. B. 86, 269-277
Bruce, D., Hamerton, A. E., Watson, D. P. & Bruce, M. E. (1914) Trypanosomes found in wild Glossina morsitans and wild game in the "fly belt" of the Upper Shire valley. Proc. R. Soc. Ser. B. 88, 39-42
Bruce, D., Harvey, D., Hamerton, A. E., Davey, J. B. & Bruce, M. E. (1915) Trypanosomes and other parasites of animals in Nyasaland. Trypanosoma cephalophi, sp. nov. Rep. sleep. Sickn. Commn. R. Soc. 16, 205-206

Buxton, P. A. (1955) The natural history of tsetse flies: an account of the biology of the genus Glossina (diptera). London School Hygiene & Tropical Medicine Memoir No. 10 London: H. K. Lewis

Caccavella, A. (1939) Nota preliminare sulle tripanosomiasi dell' occidente etiopico. Riv. Biol. colon. 2, 233-225

Camago, E. P. (1964) Growth and differentiation in Trypanosoma cruzi. I. Origin of metacyclic trypanosomes in liquid media. Revta Inst. Med. trop. S. Paulo 6, 93-100

Cardamatis, J. P. & Photinos, S. (1912) Étude biologique et histologique sur les trypanosomes chez les bovidés en Grèce. Zentbl. Bakt. ParasitKde Orig. 61, 538-542

Carini, A. (1911) Présence de trypanosomes chez les bovidés à São Paulo. Bull. Soc. Path. exot. 4, 191-192

Carmichael, J. (1926) Rinderpest serum and the pathogenicity of Trypanosoma theileri. Trans. R. Soc. trop. Med. Hyg. 20, 303-304

Carmichael, J. (1939) Turning sickness of cattle and Trypanosoma theileri. Parasitology 31, 498-500

Carpano, M. (1913) Trypanosoma tipo theileri nei bovini nella Colonia Eritrea. Clinica vet., Milano 36, 439-452 (also in Zentbl. Bakt. ParasitKde Orig. 70, 209-217)

Carpano, M. (1924) Su di un trypanosoma tipo theileri osservato nei bovini della Campagna Romana. Annali Ig. sper. 34, 169-176 + 1 plate

Carpano, M. (1932) Localisations du Trypanosoma theileri dans les organs internes des bovins. Son cycle evolutif. Annls Parasit. hum. comp. 10, 305-322 + 2 plates

Carpano, M. (1938) Sulla morfologia dei tripanosomidi in rapporto all' ambiente. Riv. Parassit. 2, 81-90 + 1 plate

Chagas, C. (1909) Ueber eine neue Trypanosomiasis des Menschen. Studien über Morphologie und Entwicklungszyklus des Schizotrypanum cruzi n. gen., n. sp., Erreger einer neuen Krankheit des Menschen. Mems. Inst. Oswaldo Cruz 1, 159-218

Christiansen, -. Quoted by Yakimoff & Kohl-Yakimoff (1911a)

Clarkson, M. J. & McCabe, W. (1970) Trypanosoma vivax in ruminants. Trans. R. Soc. trop. Med. Hyg. 64, 164-165

Coles, A. C. (1913) Trypanosoma found in a cow in England. Parasitology 5, 247-252 + 1 plate

Coles, A. C. (1914) Blood parasites found in mammals, birds and fishes in England. Parasitology 7, 17-61 + 4 plates

Crawley, H. (1909) Studies on blood and blood parasites. III. Trypanosoma americanum n. sp., a trypanosome which appears in cultures made from the blood of American cattle (preliminary notice). Bull. Bur. Anim. Ind. U. S. Dep. Agric. No. 119 (also in J. comp. Path. Ther. (1910) 23, 17-26)

Crawley, H. (1912a) The protozoan parasites of domesticated animals. Bur. Anim. Ins. U. S. Dep. Agric. Report No. 27 (for 1910)

Crawley, H. (1912b) Trypanosoma americanum, a common blood parasite of American cattle. Bull. Bur. Anim. Ind. U. S. Dep. Agric. No. 145 pp. 4-39

Cross, R. F., Redman, D. R. & Bohl, E. H. (1968) Trypanosomes associated with bovine lymphocytosis. J. Am. vet. med. Ass. 153, 571-575
Croverie, P. (1920) Trypanosoma theileri varietas somalensis chez les bovidés somaliens, considéré par rapport à la peste bovine et aux séro-vaccinations anti-pesteuses. Rev. Path. comp. 20, 183
Cunningham, M. P., Lumsden, W. H. R. & Webber, W. A. F. (1963) Preservation of viable trypanosomes in lymph tubes at low temperature. Expl Parasit. 14, 280-284
Curasson, G. (1925) Trypanosoma theileri au Soudan français. Bull. Soc. Path. exot. 18, 823-824
Curasson, G. (1943) Traité de protozoologie vétérinaire et comparée. I. Trypanosomes. Paris: Vigot Frères
Davis, B. S. (1952) Studies on the trypanosomes of some California mammals. Univ. Calif. Publ. Zool. 57, 145-230
Deane, L. M. (1961) Tripanosomideos de maniferos de Região Amazõnica. I. Alguns flagelados encontrados no sangue de mamiferos silvestres do Estado do Pará. Revta Inst. Med. trop. S. Paulo 3, 15-28
Deane, L. M. (1967) Tripanosomídeos de mamiferos da região Amazonica IV. Hemoscopia e xenodiagnostico de animais silvestres da Estrada Belem - Brasilia. Revta Inst. Med. trop. S. Paulo 9, 143-148
Deane, M. P. & Kirchner, E. (1963) Life-cycle of Trypanosoma conorhini. Influence of temperature and other factors on growth and morphogenesis. J. Protozool. 10, 391-397
Delanoe, P. (1911) Présence de trypanosomes chez les bovidés en France. Bull. Soc. Path. exot. 4, 112-116
Delpy (1931) Renseignements practiques pour l'indentification des trypanosomes des animaux en A. O. F. Recl Méd. vét. exot., Ec. Alfort 4, 31-40
Diaz-Ungria, C., Maldonado, C. & Colina, E. S. (1969) Nota previa sobre el hallazgo del Trypanosoma theileri en bovinos de Venezuela. Revta vet. Venez. 26, 152-154
Dios, R. & Zuccarini, J. A. (1924) Première constatation de la trypanosomiase bovine en République Argentine. C. r. Séanc. Soc. Biol. 91, 23-24
Dikmans, G., Manthei, C. A. & Frank, A. H. (1957) Demonstration of Trypanosoma theileri in the stomach of an aborted bovine fetus. Cornell Vet. 47, 344-353
Djatkova, I. (1937) [A case of trypanosomiasis in a cow in Yugoslavia.] Jugosl. vet. Glasn. 17, 57-60
Dodd, S. (1912) Trypanosoma ingens in the mouse deer (Tragulus javanicus). J. comp. Path. Ther. 25, 281-285
Drachinskii, S. I. & Markov, A. A. (1927) [Geographical distribution of the bovine trypanosome, Tr. theileri, in the U. S. S. R.] Trudy gos. Inst. eksp. Vet. 4, No. 2 pp. 120-123
Dschunkowsky, E. & Luhs, J. (1909) Protozoan diseases of domestic animals in Transcaucasia. Trans. IXth int. vet. Congr., The Hague Vol. I. pp. 43-47

Dudukalov, A. A. (1908) [The trypanosomes of cattle. Preliminary report.] Russk. Vrach. 7, 410-411
Dudukalov, A. A. & Dudukalova, N. (1910) Ob iskusstvennom kultivirovanii tripanozom naidennykh u nogatago skota. Sooschenie vtoroe. Arkh. vet. Nauk. 40, 1-4
Duke, H. L. (1912) Antelope and their relation to trypanosomiasis. Proc. R. Soc. Ser. B. 85, 156-169
Durrant & Holmes, J. D. E. (1904) A trypanosoma found in blood of cattle in India. J. comp. Path. Ther. 17, 209-210
Dutton, J. E., Todd, J. L. & KINGHORN, A. (1907) Cattle trypanosomiasis in the Congo Free State. Ann. trop. Med. Parasit. 1, 233-271
Dutton, J. E., Todd, J. L. & Tobey, E. N. (1906) Concerning certain parasitic protozoa observed in Africa. Part I. Mem. Lpool Sch. trop. Med. 21 pp. 87-97
Egypt (1942) Annual report of the Veterinary Services
Ewing, S. A. & Carnahan, D. L. (1967) Occurrence of Trypanosoma theileri in bovine peripheral blood. J. Am. vet. med. Ass. 150, 1131-1132
Ezzart, A. M. E. (1961) Protozoal diseases of veterinary importance in Egypt. Progress in protozoology, pp. 478-481 Prague: Czechoslovak Academy of Sciences
Falshaw, P. S. & Lingard, A. (1907) A note on a new species of trypanosoma discovered in the blood of an Indian bullock at Singapre. J. trop. vet. Sci. 2, 217-220 + 1 plate
F. A. O. (1968) Animal health yearbook for 1967. Rome: F. A. O.
Ferreira, F. S. da C. (1948) As tripanosomiases nos teritorios Africanos Portugueses. Africa Ocidental (Angola e Guine). Africa Oriental (Mocambique). Lisboa pp. 52
Florinsky, -. (1928) Quoted by Sprinholz-Schmidt (1938)
Flu, P. C. (1908) Über die Flagellaten im Darm von Melophagus ovinus. Arch. Protistenk. 12, 147-153
Folkers, C. & Mohammed, A. N. (1965) The importance of biting flies other than Glossina in the epidemiology of trypanosomiasis in cattle in Shika - Northern Nigeria. Bull. epizoot. Dis. Afr. 13, 331-339
Frank, G. (1909) Über den Befund von Trypanosomen bei einem in Stein-Wingert (Westerwald, Regierungsbezirk Wiesbaden) verendeten Rinde. Z. InfektKrankh. parasit. Krankh. Hyg. Haustiere 5, 313-315
Frank, G. & Frosch, P. (1909) Über die Bedeutung des Befundes rinderpathogener Trypanosomen in Deutschland. Z. InfektKrankh. parasit. Krankh. Hyg. Haustiere 5, 330-334
Fraser, A. D. & Duke, H. L. (1912) The relation of wild animals to trypanosomiasis. Rep. sleep. sickn. Commn. R. Soc. 12, 26-36
Frosch, P. (1909) Ätiologische Ermittelungen über das Trypanosoma frank. Z. InfektKrankh. parasit. Krankh. Hyg. Haustiere 5, 316-329
Gaiger, S. H. (1910) Further observations on trypanosomiasis. J. trop. vet. Sci. 6, 21-43
Galliard, H. (1925) Sur un cas d'infection à Trypanosoma theileri et Piroplasma bigeminum. Annls Parasit. hum. comp. 3, 21-27

Gallo, P. (1938) Le tripanosomiasi animali nel Nicaragua. Archo, ital. Sci. med. colon. 19, 344-349
Glaser, R. W. (1922) A study of Trypanosoma americanum. J. Parasit. 8, 136-144
Glover, P. E. (1961) The tsetse problem in Northern Nigeria. Nairobi: Patwa News Agency
Godfrey, D. G., Killick-Kendrick, R. & Ferguson, W. (1965) Bovine trypanosomiasis in Nigeria. IV. Observations on cattle trekked along a trade-route through areas infested with tsetse fly. Ann. trop. Med. Parasit. 59, 255-269
Gray, A. R. & Nixon, J. (1967) Observations on the incidence and importance of Trypanosoma theileri in Nigeria. Ann. trop. Med. Parasit. 61, 251-260
Hadwen, S. (1912) Quoted by Wenyon (1926)
Hall, O. (1953) Trypanosomiasis. Rep. Vet. Direct. Gen., Canada 1951-2 p. 11
Hamerton, A. E. (1911) An experiment to ascertain at what point on the road between Kavirondo and Uganda, cattle become infected with trypanosomes. An account of a journey from Kisumu to Jinja. Rep. sleep. Sickn. Commn R. Soc. 11, 271-275
Hare, W. C. D. & Soulsby, E. J. L. (1969) Stimulation of DNA synthesis in bovine leukocyte cultures by Trypanosoma theileri antigen. J. Parasit. 55, 973-976
Hare, W. C. D., Yang, T.-J. & McFeely, R. A. (1967) A survey of chromosome findings in 47 cases of bovine lymphosarcoma (leukemia). J. natn. Cancer Inst. 38, 383-392
Harley, J. M. B. (1963) Diagnosis of trypanosomiasis in a herd of cattle. Rep. E. Afr. Trypan. Res. Org., 1962-3 pp. 12-13
Hartmann, M. & Nöller, W. (1918) Untersuchungen über die Cytologie von Trypanosoma theileri. Arch. Protistenk. 38, 355-373
Haughwout, F. G. & Youngberg, S. (1920) A trypanosoma associated with a fatal disease in the carabao. Philipp. J. Sci. 16, 75-85
Heanley, C. M. (1908) A note on the occurrence of a large trypanosome in the blood of native in South-China. J. comp. Path. Ther. 21, 178-179
Herbert, I. V. (1961) Bovine trypanosomiasis due to Trypanosoma theileri Laveran, 1902 and its occurrence in Eire. Irish vet. J. 15, 230-236
Herbert, I. V. (1962) Studies on the in vitro cultivation of trypanosomes with special reference to Trypanosoma theileri Laveran, 1902. Ann. appl. Biol. 50, 354-355
Herbert, I. V. (1964) Trypanosoma theileri, Laveran, 1902. A cosmopolitan parasite of cattle. Vet. Bull., Weybridge 34, 563-570
Herbert, I. V. (1965a) Cytochemistry of in vitro cultured Trypanosoma theileri. Expl Parasit. 16, 348-362
Herbert, I. V. (1965b) Cytoplasmic inclusions and organelles of in vitro cultured Trypanosoma theileri and Trypanosoma melophagium and some speculations on their function. Expl. Parasit. 17, 24-40

Herbert, I. V. (1965c) Some observations on the isolation and in vitro culture of two mammalian trypanosomes, Trypanosoma theileri Laveran, 1902, and T. melophagium Flu, 1908, with special reference to T. theileri. Ann. trop. Med. Parasit. 59, 277-293

Hoare, C. A. (1923) An experimental study of the sheep-trypanosome (T. melophagium Flu, 1908) and its transmission by the sheep-ked (Melophagus ovinus L.). Parasitology 15, 365-424 + 4 plates

Hoare, C. A. (1929) Some blood protozoa from Uganda. Trans. R. Soc. trop. Med. Hyg. 23, 327-328

Hoare, C. A. (1936) Morphological and taxonomic studies on mammalian trypanosomes. I. Parasitology 28, 98-109

Hoare, C. A. (1949) Handbook of medical protozoology. London: Baillière, Tindall & Cox

Hoare, C. A. (1957) The classification of trypanosomes of veterinary and medical importance. Vet. Rev. Annot. 3, 1-13

Hoare, C. A. (1964) Morphological and taxonomic studies on mammalian trypanosomes. X. Revision of the systematics. J. Protozool. 11, 200-207

Hoare, C. A. (1966) The classification of mammalian trypanosomes. Ergebn. Mikrobiol. ImmunForsch. exp. Ther. 39, 43-57

Hoare, C. A. & Wallace, F. G. (1966) Development stages of trypanosomatid flagellates: a new terminology. Nature, Lond. 212, 1385-1386

Holmes, J. D. E. (1904) Some diseases complicating rinderpest among cattle of India. J. comp. Path. Ther. 17, 317-326

Honigberg, B. M., Balamuth, W., Bovee, E. C., Corliss, J. O., Gojdics, M., Hall, R. P., Kudo, R. R., Levine, N. D., Loeblich, A. R. Jr., Weiser, J. & Wenrich, D. H. (1964) A revised classification of the phylum Protozoa. J. Protozool. 11, 7-20

Hornby, H. E. (1930) Control of animal trypanosomiasis. XIth Int. vet. Congr. London 1930 pp. 614-631

Hornby, H. E. (1936) Trypanosomiasis and tsetse fly. Ann. Rep. Dep. Vet. Sci. Anim. Husb., Tanganyika, 1935 pp. 13-14

Hornby, H. E. (1949) Animal trypanosomiasis in Eastern Africa. London: H. M. Stat. Off.

Hornby, H. E. & Bailey, H. W. (1929) Research on trypanosomiasis. Ann. Rep. Dep. Vet. Sci. Anim. Husb., Tanganyika 1928 pp. 27-28

Hornby, H. E., Evans, S. A. & Cornell, R. L. (1934) Pathogenicity of Trypanosoma theileri. Ann. Rep. Dep. Vet. Sci. Anim. Husb., Tanganyika 1933 pp. 34-36

India (1940) Agriculture and animal husbandry in India 1937 - 1938. Delhi: Imperial Council of Agricultural Research

Iwata, A., Takamura, M., Kita, E., Inui, S., Kawashima, H. & Nagai, H. (1959) [On the trypanosome isolated from severely anaemic cows. A case of mixed infection with a small piroplasm.] J. Jap. vet. med. Ass. 12, 22-28

Jegen, G. (1924) Die protozoäre Parasitenfauna der Stechfliege, Stomoxys calcitrans. Ein Beitrag zur Erforschung parasitischer Protozoen in den blutsaugenden insekten. Zool. Jb. Abt. Anat. 46, 389-472

Johns, F. M. (1913) On the adult forms of _Trypanosoma americanum_ in naturally infected animals. Am. J. trop. Dis. _1_, 49-57
Johns, F. M. (1914) _Trypanosoma americanum._ New Orl. med. surg. J. _66_, 533-534
Julian, R. J. (1971) The isolation of trypanosomes from cattle in Ontario. Can. J. comp. Med. _35_, 192-194
Kawamura, -. (1916) Quoted by Saisawa _et al._ (1933)
Kearney, W. (1926) Report of the veterinary pathologist for the period October 1924 - December 1925. Ann. Rep. Vet. Dep. N. Prov., Nigeria
Kehoe, D. (1916) Laboratory records; Research laboratory, Division of veterinary education and research; Pietermaritzburg, Natal (Reported by Robinson, E. M. (1923) in S. Afr. J. Sci. _20_, 432-436)
Kelser, R. A. (1927) Transmission of surra among animals of the equine species. Philipp. J. Sci. _34_, 115-139
Kenya (1957 & 1958) Ann. Rep. Vet. Dep.
Kerr, W. R. (1942/3) Trichomoniasis in the bull. Vet. J. _98_, 209-217 & _99_, 4-8
Kerr, W. R. & Robertson, M. (1943) A study of the antibody response of cattle to _Trichomonas foetus._ J. comp. Path. Ther. _53_, 280-297
Keymer, I. F. (1967) _Trypanosoma (Megatrypanum)_ spp. Hoare, 1964 of ruminants. Vet. Rec. _80_, 286
Keymer, I. F. (1969) Investigations on the duiker (_Sylvicarpa grimmia_) and its blood protozoa in Central Africa. Phil. Trans. R. Soc. Ser. B. _255_, 33-108
Kinghorn, A. & Yorke, W. (1912) Further observations on the trypanosomes of game and domestic stock in North-Eastern Rhodesia. Ann. trop. Med. Parasit. _6_, 483-493
Kinghorn, A., Yorke, W. & Lloyd, L. (1913) Final report of the Luangwa sleeping sickness commission of the British South Africa Company, 1911 - 1912. Ann. trop. Med. Parasit. _7_, 183-302
Kleine, F. K. (1910) Trypanosomenbefunde am Tanganyika und andere Beobachtungen. Dt. med. Wschr. _36_, 1400-1402
Kleine, F. K. & Fischer, W. (1912) Die rolle der Säugetiere bei der Verbreitung der Schlafkrankheit und Trypanosomenbefunde bei Säugetieren am Tanganyika. Z. Hyg. InfektKrankh. _70_, 1-23
Knuth, P. (1909) Über die Morphologie des _Trypanosoma frank._ Z. InfektKrankh. Parasit. Krankh. Hyg. Haustiere _6_, 39-45
Knuth, P. (1910) Über die in deutschen Rindern gefundenen Trypanosomen. Berl. tierärztl. Wschr. _26_, 810-811
Knuth, P. & Rauchbaar, G. (1910a) Weitere Nachforschungen nach Trypanosomen beim Rinde in Kreise Oberwesterwald nebst einem Beitrag zur Kenntnis der in deutschen Stechfliegen (spezies: _Tabanus_ und _Haematopota_) parasitierenden Flagellaten. Z. InfektKrankh. parasit. Krankh. Hyg. Haustiere _8_, 140-154
Knuth, P. & Rauchbaar, G. (1910b) Zum Vorkommen von Trypanosomen bei Rindern in Deutschland. Berl. tierärztl. Wschr. _26_, 609-610

Knuth, P., Rauchbaar, G. & Morgenstern, P. (1910) Nachweis von Trypanosomen beim Rinde im Kreise Oberwesterwald mittelst Züchtung in Blut-Bouillon. Berl. tierärztl. Wschr. 26, 539-540

Koch, R. (1904) Über die Trypanosomenkrankheiten. Dt. med. Wschr. 30, 1705-1710 (also in Br. med. J. (1904) 2, 1445-1449)

Kohl-Yakimoff, N., Yakimoff, W. L. & Bekensky, P. W. (1913a) Le trypanosome des bovidés (Tr. theileri ou du type voisin) en Russie d''Europe. Bull. Soc. Path. exot. 6, 433-434

Kohl-Yakimoff, N., Yakimoff, W. L. & Schokhor, N. J. (1913b) Le trypanosome des bovidés (Tr. theileri ou du type voisin) au Turkestan. Bull. Soc. Path. exot. 6, 434

Kränzle (1912) Trypanosomen im Blute einer Kuh. Munch. tierärztl. Wschr. 56, 925

Kraneveld, F. C. (1931) Enkele overbrengingsproeven van Trypanosoma theileri Laveran 1902 met Tabaniden. Ned. Indische Bl. Diergeneesk. 43, 132-192

Kraneveld, F. C. & Djaendedin, R. (1932) Het Voorkomen van met Trypanosoma theileri Laveran 1902 in Nederlandsch-Indië. Ned. Indische Bl. Diergeneesk. 44, 207-215

Kusel, J. P., Moore, K. E. & Weber, M. M. (1967) The ultrastructure of Crithidia fasciculata and morphological changes induced by growth in acriflavin. J. Protozool. 14, 283-296

Kuttler, K. L., Adams, L. G. & Zaraza, H. (1969) An epizootiological and geographic survey of Anaplasma marginale and Trypanosoma theileri in Colombia. A. V. M. A. Convention, Minneapolis, Minnesota

Lamy, L. & Bouley, G. (1967) Observation en France, chez un veau, d'un cas d'infection massive à Trypanosoma theileri, Laveran 1902. Bull. Acad. vét. Fr. 40, 323-325

Lanham, S. H. (1968) The separation of trypanosomes from blood cells and their behaviour on TEAE- and DEAE-cellulose and on DEAE-Sephadex. Trans. R. Soc. trop. Med. Hyg. 62, 129-130

Lanham, S. M. (1970) The separation of stercorarian trypanosomes from infected blood using DEAE-cellulose. XI seminar on trypanosomiasis research. Overseas Development Ministry, London

Laveran, A. (1902a) Sur un nouveau trypanosome des bovidés (Trypanosoma theileri). C. r. hebd. Séanc. Acad. Sci., Paris 134, 512-514

Laveran, A. (1902b) Au sujet de deux trypanosomes des bovidés du Transvaal. C. r. hebd. Séanc. Acad. Sci., Paris 135, 717-721

Laveran, M. A. (1903) Sur deux hippobosques du Transvaal susceptibles de propager Trypanosoma theileri. C. r. Séanc. Soc. Biol. 55, 242-243

Leach, T. M. (1964) Ann. Rep. Nigerian Inst. Trypan. Res., 1964 pp. 22-23 & 35-36

Leach, T. M. (1965) Ann. Rep. Nigerian Inst. Trypan. Res., 1965

Legrain, -. (1896) In "Nouvelles et informations" Recl. Med. vet. Ec. Alfort, 15th April, 266 (quoting from Le Progress Veterinaire 15th March, 1896)

Levine, N. D., Watrach, A. M., Kantor, S. & Hardenbrook, H. J. (1956) A case of bovine trypanosomiasis due to Trypanosoma theileri in Illinois. J. Parasit. 42, 553
Lingard, A. (1903) The giant trypanosoma discovered in the blood of bovines. Zentbl. Bakt. ParasitKde. I. Abt. 35, 234-238
Lingard, A. (1904) A short account of the various trypanosomata found to date in India in the blood of some of the lower animals and fish. Indian med. Gaz. 445
Lingard, A. (1907) Different species of trypanosomata observed in bovines in India. J. trop. vet. Sci. 2, 4-51
Lühe, M. (1906) Die im blute schmarotzenden Protozoen und ihre nächsten Verwandten. In "Handbuch der tropen - Krankheiten", edited by C. Mense, Vol. 3, pp. 69-268 Leipzig
Lühs, F. (1905) Trypanosoma theileri in Transkaukasien. Archs. Parasit. 10, 171-186 + 2 plates
Lundholm, B. D., Storz, J. & McKercher, D. G. (1959) Trypanosoma theileri as a contaminant of tissue origin in cultures of fetal bovine kidney cells in vitro. Virology 8, 394-396
Macfie, J. W. S. (1913) Trypanosomiasis of domestic animals in Northern Nigeria. Ann. trop. Med. Parasit. 7, 1-20
Mackie, F. P. (1911) Report on an outbreak of disease among cattle on the estate of A. B. Walsh, Esq., at Kabula Muliro. Rep. sleep. Sickn. Commn. R. Soc. 11, 264-268
Mahajan, M. R. (1939) Surra in Hyderbad State. Indian J. vet. Sci. 9, 217-221 + 2 plates
Malbrant, R., Bayrou, M. & Rapin, P. (1939) Protozooses sanguines des animaux domestique en Afrique équatoriale française. Bull. Soc. Path. exot. 32, 953-960
Maliavkine, -. (1926) Quoted by Sprinholz-Schmidt (1938)
Malmquist, W. A. (1965) Trypanosomes in leucocyte cultures. Vet. Rec. 77, 350
Manceaux, L., Yakimoff, W. L. & Kohl-Yakimoff, N. (1911a) Culture et morphologie du trypanosome type theileri des boeufs tunisiens. Bull. Soc. Path. exot. 4, 378-380
Manceaux, L., Yakimoff, W. L. & Kohl-Yakimoff, N. (1911b) Recherches sur les trypanosomes du genre "theileri" des bovides en Tunisie. Deuxième note. Culture et morphologie des trypanosomes normaux des bovidés tunisiens. Archs. Inst. Pasteur Tunis 6, 262-267
Martini, E. (1909) The development of a piroplasma and trypanosoma of cattle in artificial culture medium. Philipp. J. Sci. Ser. B. 4, 147-170
Marzinowsky, -. (1911) Quoted by Sprinholz-Schmidt (1938)
Mayer, M. (1909) Über Trypanosoma theileri und diesem verwandte Rindertrypanosomen. Z. InfektKrankh. parasit. krankh. Hyg. Haustiere 6, 46-51
Mayer, M. (1912) Pathogen Trypanosomen. In "Handbuch der pathogen. protozoen", edited by von Prowazek, S. and W. Nöller, Vol. 1, p. 299 Leipzig

Mazza, S., Romaña, C. & Fiora, A. (1932) Algunos hemoparasitos de mamiferos del norte. 7th Reun. Soc. Argent. Patol. Reg. Norte, Buenos Aires Part 2, pp. 990-997
Mendes, A. C., Mora, A. D., Monteiro, A. S. & Bruto da Costa, B. (1909) La maladie du somneil à l'Ile du Prince. Archos Hyg. Patol. exot., Lisb. 2, 275-350
Mesnil, M. (1913) Abstract of paper by K. J. Wrublewski (1912) Bull. Inst. Pasteur, Paris 11, 292
Mesnil, M. (1923) Abstract of paper by O. Trautmann (1922) Bull. Inst. Pasteur, Paris 21, 465-466
Mikačić, D. (1941) Parasitska fauna naseg goveda. Vet. Arhiv. 11, 28-50
Miyajima, M. (1907) On the cultivation of a bovine piroplasma: a preliminary communication. Philipp. J. Sci. Ser. B. 2, 83-92
Molyneux, D. H. (1968) The ultrastructure of Trypanosoma lewisi in the rectum of Nosopsyllus fasciatus. Trans. R. Soc. trop. Med. Hyg. 62, 6-7
Molyneux, D. H. (1969) The attachment of Trypanosoma lewisi in the rectum of its vector flea Nosopsyllus fasciatus. Trans. R. Soc. trop. Med. Hyg. 63, 117
Montgomery, R. E. & Kinghorn, A. (1908) A report on trypanosomiasis of domestic stock in Northern-Western Rhodesia. Ann. trop. Med. Parasit. 2, 97-132
Mornet, M. (1941) Sur les parasites sanguicoles des animaux domestique au Niger. Bull. Servs zootech. Epizoot. Afr. occid. fr. 4, 92-97
Morris, D. (1965) The mammals. London: Hodder & Stoughton
Morris, K. R. S. (1932) Trypanosomes of game in the Gold Coast. W. Afr. Med. J. 5, 65-67
Morriss, -. (1940) Personal communication quoted by Curasson (1943)
Mulhearn, C. R. (1942) Unpublished information quoted by Seddon (1952)
Nabarro, D. & Greig, E. D. W. (1905) Trypanosomata found in the lower animals in Uganda and East Africa. Rep. sleep. Sickn. Commn. R. Soc. 5, 18
Naik, -. (1937) Quoted by Sarwar (1937)
Neitz, W. O. (1931) Blood parasites of game in Zululand. Preliminary report. 17th Rep. Dir. vet. Serv. Anim. Ind., S. Afr. pp. 45-60
Neitz, W. O. (1933) Blood parasites of game in Zululand. Further report. Onderstepoort J. vet. Sci. 1, 411-417
Neveu-Lemaire, M. (1943) Traité de protozoologie medicale et vététinaire. p. 807 Paris: Vigot Frères
Newton, B. A. (1971) DNA of stercorarian trypanosomes. Trans. R. Soc. trop. Med. Hyg. 65, 425-426
Nieschulz, O. (1931) Ueber Darmflagellaten con Tabaniden in Java. Z. ParasitKde 3, 267-268
Nigeria (1927) Annual Report of the Veterinary Department, Northern Provinces 1927
Nigeria (1950 & 1951) Annual reports of the Veterinary Department for 1949-50 and 1950-1

Nöller, W. (1916) Die Übertragung des Trypanosoma theileri Laveran, 1902. Berl. tierärztl. Wschr. 32, 457-460

Nöller, W. (1917) Blut- und Insektenflagellatenzuchtung auf Platten. Arch. Schiffs- u. Tropenhyg. 21, 59-94

Nöller, W. (1920) Neure Forschungen auf dem Gebiete der Trypanosomen-züchtung. Arch. Schiffs- u. Tropenhyg. 24, 168-172

Nöller, W. (1925) Der Nachweis des Überträgers des gemeinen Rindertrypanosomas T. theilieri mit Hilfe des Kulturverfahrens. Zentbl. Bakt. ParasitKde 79, 133-142

Nöller, W. (1931) Die nächsten Verwandten der Blutflagellaten und ihre Beziehungen zu den Blutbewohnenden Formen. In "Handbuch der pathogen protozoen", edited by S. von Prowazek & W. Noller, Vol. 3, pp. 1893-1906 Leipzig

Novy, F. G. & MacNeal, W. J. (1904) On the cultivation of Trypanosoma brucei. J. inf. Dis. 1, 1-30

Nyasaland (1955 - 1960) Annual reports of the Department of Veterinary Services and Animal Industry.

O'Farrell, W. R. (1913) Hereditary infection, with special reference to its occurrence in Hyalomma aegyptium infected with Crithidia hyalommae. Ann. trop. Med. Parasit. 7, 545-562

Old, J. E. S. (1915) Report on certain investigations in the elephant marsh; Ruo district. Rep. sleep. Sickn. Commn. R. Soc. 16, 210-212

Onyango, R. J. (1967) Rep. E. Afr. Trypan. Res. Org., 1966 pp. 28, 62-64 & 79-80

Packchanian, A. A. (1934) On the cultivation of seven species of trypanosomes in vitro. Science 80, 407-408

Packchanian, A. A. (1943) On the viability of various species of Trypanosoma and Leishmania cultures. J. Parasit. 29, 275-277

Packchanian, A. A. (1957) The isolation and cultivation of hemo-flagellates in pure culture from six species of insects. Tex. Rep. Biol. Med. 15, 399-410

Page, W. A. (in press) Feeding behaviour and trypanosomatid infections of some tabanids and Culicidae (Diptera) in Colombia.

Panama (1941) Annual report of the Gorgas Memorial Laboratory, Washington, DC. 1940

Panse, O. (1904) Trypanosoma theileri (?) in Deutsch-Ostafrika. Z. Hyg. InfektKrankh. 5, 376-378

Paratschouk, -. (1924) Quoted by Sprinholz-Schmidt (1938)

Parzwanidze, -. (1925) Quoted by Sprinholz-Schmidt (1938)

Patton, W. S. (1909) The life-cycle of a species of Crithidia parasitic in the intestinal tracts of Tabanus hilarius and Tabanus sp. Arch. Protistenk. 15, 333-362

Pease, H. T. (1909) Trypanosoma theileri and galziekte. J. trop. vet. Sci. 4, 532-539

Peter, O. (1910) Morphologische und experimentelle Studien über ein neues, bei Rindern in Uruguay (Südamerika) gefundenes Trypanosoma. Arch. Schiffs- u. Tropenhyg. 14, 7-40 + 1 plate

Pifano, F. (1941) Parasitismo natural de Amblyomma longyrostre Koch, 1844 por Schizotrypanum cruzi Chagas, 1909. Gaceta Med. Caracas 48, 288-289
Rao, M. A. N. & Ayyar, L. S. P. (1931) Some observations on trypanosomiasis in Madras presidency. Indian vet. J. 8, 111-118
Refik Bey (1902) Modifications leucocytaires dans la bovine. Ann. Inst. Pasteur 16, 163-168
Reichenow, E. (1940) Ostafrikanische Beobachtungen am Trypanosomiden. Arch. Protistenk. 94, 267-287
Reid, H. W., Burridge, M. J., Pullan, N. B., Sutherst, R. W. & Wain, E. B. (1966) Stercorarian trypanosomes in cattle and wild animals in East Africa - preliminary report. 11th Meet. Int. sci. Counc. Trypanosomiasis Res. pp. 49-50
Reid, H. W., Burridge, M. J., Pullan, N. B., Sutherst, R. W. & Wain, E. B. (1970) Survey for trypanosome infections in domestic cattle and wild animals in areas of East Africa. IV. Stercorarian trypanosome infections in cattle and wild animals in East Africa. Br. vet. J. 126, 642-647
Richardson, U. F. (1930) Trypanosome cultures. Rep. vet. Dep. Uganda, 1929 pp. 11-12
Richardson, U. F. (1948) Veterinary protozoology. Edinburgh: Oliver & Boyd
Ristic, M. & Trager, W. (1958) Cultivation at 37°C of a trypanosome (Trypanosoma theileri) from cows with depressed milk production. J. Protozool. 5, 146-148
Robertson, M. (1956) Some aspects of trypanosomiasis with particular reference to the work of Sir David Bruce. J. trop. Med. Hyg. 59, 67-77
Robinson, E. M. (1923) A note on the cultivation of flagellates of the Trypanosoma theileri type from the blood of South African cattle. S. Afr. J. Sci. 20, 432-436
Robinson, G. (1929) Rep. Med. Sanit. Dep., Gold Coast 1928-1929 pp. 76-78
Rodhain, J. (1916) Note sur les trypanoses et les piroplasmoses des grands animaux de l'Ouellé. Bull. Soc. Path. exot. 9, 95-109
Rodhain, J., Pons, C., Vandenbranden, F. & Bequaert, J. (1912) Les trypanoses animales au Bas-Katanga et leurs rapports avec les glossines (deuxieme note). Bull. Soc. Path. exot. 5, 281-287
Rodhain, J., Pons, C., Vandenbranden, F. & Bequaert, J. (1913) Rapport sur les travaux de la mission scientifique du Katanga (octobre, 1910 à septembre 1912). Bruxelles: Hayez, Imprimeur de l'Academie Royale
Roetti, C. (1940) Sull' esistenza di un Tripanosoma del tipo theileri nei dromedari somali. Ann. Pat. trop. Parasit. 1, 295-297
Sadowsky, -. (1910) Quoted by Sprinholz-Schmidt (1938)
Saisawa, K., Taise, K. -I. & Kaneko, K. (1933) Study on Trypanosoma theileri. Jap. J. exp. Med. 11, 101-105 + 1 plate
Sasaki, N. & Nishi, T. (1950) [On Trypanosoma theileri collected from cattle in the Tokachi District, Hokkaido.] J. Jap. vet. med. Ass. 3, 350-352 [Ja]

Sassouchin, -. & Matwejeff, -. (1922) Quoted by Sprinholz-Schmidt (1938)
Schaudinn, F. (1904) Generations- und Wirtswechsel bei Trypanosoma und Spirochaete (vorläufige mitteilung). Arb. K. GesundhAmt. 20, 387-489
Schein, H. (1907) Hématozoaires des bovidés en Indo-Chine. Annls Inst. Pasteur, Paris 21, 660-665 (English translation in J. trop. vet. Sci. 3, 202-206)
Schilling, C. (1903) On nagana and other trypanosomes. J. trop. Med. 6, 45-47
Schmid, F. (1938) Trypanosomen bei einer milzbrandverdächtigen Kuh. Münch. tierärztl. Wschr. 89, 25-26
Schmitt, F. M. (1910) Zum Vorkommen von Trypanosomen vom Typus des T. theileri in deutschen Rindern. Berl. tierärztl. Wschr. 26, 841-842
Schmitt, F. M. (1911) Trypanosomen und Babesien in deutschen Rindern. Berl. tierärztl. Wschr. 27, 207-208
Schoenbeck, K. (1910) Beobachtungen eines anscheinend pathogenen zur Gruppe des Trypanosoma theileri gehörigen Trypanosoma in Deutsch-Ostafrika, zugleich ein Beitrag zur Behandlung und Prophylaxe der Trypanose. Arch. Schiffs- u. Tropenhyg. 14, 548-550
Schoening, H. W. (1925) Complement fixation tests on serums of cattle harboring Trypanosoma americanum. Am. J. trop. Med. 5, 247-249
Schwetz, J. (1927) Notes sur les trypanosomiases animales du Haut-Katanga. Annls. Soc. belge Méd. trop. 7, 135-149
Schwetz, J. (1928) Notes sur les trypanosomiases animales de Stanleyville. Bull. agric. Congo belge 19, 562-576
Schwetz, J. (1930) Sur un cas d'infection intense par Trypanosoma theileri. Annls Parasit. hum. comp. 8, 135-139
Schwetz, J. (1931) Notes morphologiques sur les trypanosomoses animales de Stanleyville et du Congo Oriental. Annls. Parasit. hum. comp. 9, 392-422
Sergent, Ed. & Sergent, Et. (1911) Présence de trypanosomes chez les bovidés en Algérie. Bull. Soc. Path. exot. 4, 40-42
Sergent, E., Donatien, A., Parrot, L. & Lestoquard, F. (1945) Études sur les piroplasmoses bovines. pp. 257-258 Alger: Institut Pasteur
Simpson, C. F. & Green, J. H. (1959) Cultivation of Trypanosoma theileri in liquid medium at 37°C. Cornell Vet. 49, 102-193
Simpson, C. F. & Sanders, D. A. (1951) Anaplasmosis in cattle. Rep. Fla agric. Exp. Stn pp. 114-115
Sollod, A. E. & Soulsby, E. J. L. (1968) Cultivation of Trypanosoma theileri at 37°C in partially defined media. J. Protozool. 15, 463-466
Splitter, E. J. & Soulsby, E. J. L. (1967) Isolation and continuous cultivation of Trypanosoma theileri in media containing tissue culture fluids. Expl Parasit. 21, 137-148
Splitter, E. J., Soulsby, E. J. L., Williams, J. F. & Jeska, E. L. (1967) Gel-diffusion and hemagglutination studies with Trypanosoma theileri. Expl Parasit. 20, 160-166

Sprinholz-Schmidt, A. J. (1938) Infection simultanée par le Trypanosoma theileri et le Theileria sergenti en Extrême-Orient. Annls. Parasit. hum. comp. 16, 117-120
Stirnimann, J. (1947) Trypanosoma theileri bei einer Kuh. Schweizer Arch. Tierheilk. 89, 140-141
Stockman, S. (1910) Preliminary note on a trypanosome of British cattle. J. comp. Path. Ther. 23, 189-192
Stolnikov, V. I. (1911) [Trypanosomiases of cattle in the European Soviet Russia.] Vest. obshch. Vet., S.-Peterb. 23, 5-13
Stolowsky, -. (1908) T. theileri im südlichen DeutschlOstafrika. Arch. Schiffs- u. Tropenhyg. 12, 30
Sudachenkov, V. V. (1931) [The geographical distribution of Trypanosoma theileri in Siberia.] Trop. Med. i Vet. Moskva 9, 275-276
Swellengrebel, N. H. (1911a) Over trypanosomen uit het bloed van Nederlandsche runderen. Tijdschr. Veeartsenijk. Veeteelt 38, 766-770
Swellengrebel, N. H. (1911a) Présence de trypanosomes chez les bovidés en Hollande. Bull. Soc. Path. exot. 4, 536-539
Tanganyika (1950-53) Annual reports of the Veterinary Department
Teague, O. & Clark, H. C. (1918) A trypanosome of Panamanian cattle and a method for concentrating trypanosomes in peripheral blood. J. infect. Dis. 22, 154-158
Tendeiro, J. (1945) Hemo-parasites da Guiné Portuguesa. (Nota prévia) Revta Med. vet., Lisb. 40, 396-402
Tendeiro, J. (1947) Tripanosomiases animais da Guiné Portuguesa. Boln cult. Guiné port. 5, 111-172
Tendeiro, J. (1949) Tripanosomiases animais da Guiné Portuguesa. Mems Cent. Estud. Guiné port. No. 10 pp. 182-204
Theiler, A. (1903) A new trypanosome and the disease caused by it in South Africa. J. comp. Path. Ther. 16, 193-216
Theiler, A. (1909) The prophylaxis of tropical and sub-tropical diseases of domesticated stock. IXth Int. vet. Congr., The Hague
Theiler, A. (1910) Gall sickness of South Africa (anaplasmosis of cattle). J. comp. Path. Ther. 23, 98-115
Thiroux, A., Wurtz, R. & Teppaz, A. (1908) Sur la maladie du sommeil et les trypanosomiases animales à la Petite Côte et dans la région des Niayes au Sénégal. Bull. Soc. Path. exot. 1, 269-273
Thomas, A. D. & Neitz, W. O. (1933) The importance of disease in wild animals. S. Afr. J. Sci. 30, 419-425
Thomson, J. D. (1908) Quoted by Hoare (1923)
Thomson, J. G. (1931) Trypanosoma tragelaphi (Kinghorn, Yorke, and Lloyd, 1913) from the blood of the humped zebu (Bos indicus) in Nigeria. Trans. R. Soc. trop. Med. 25, 5-6
Thomson, J. G. (1933) The natural occurrence of flagellates of the sub-genus Strigomonas M. and A. Lwoff in the gut of Tabanus africanus from Nyasaland and Lucilia serricata in England. J. trop. Med. Hyg. 36, 361-365

Tobie, E. J., von Brand, T. & Mehlman, B. (1950) Cultural and physiological observations on Trypanosoma rhodesiense and Trypanosoma gambiense. J. Parasit. 36, 48-54

Touré, S. M. (1968) Description complémentaire de Trypanosoma theileri Laveran, 1902. Mention particulière de formes observées en Casamance (Rép. du Sénégal). Revue Elev. Méd. vét. Pays trop. 21, 365-373

Trautmann, O. (1922) Über das kulturelle und serologische Verhalten des Trypanosoma theileri. Inaug. Diss., Tierärztl. Hochschule, Berlin (Abstr. in Bull. Inst. Past., Paris (1923) 21, 465-466)

Travassos Santos Dias, J. A. (1960) Trypanosomes found in antelopes of a region infested by Glossina austeni Newstead, 1912, in Mozambique. VIIIth Meet. int. sci. Comm. Trypan. Res. 175-177

Turner, A. W. & Murname, D. (1930a) A preliminary note on the occurrence of Trypanosoma theileri in the blood of cattle in Victoria. Aust. J. exp. Biol. med. Sci. 7, 9-11

Turner, A. W. & Murname, D. (1930b) Trypanosomes in the blood of Victorian animals. Paper 1. A preliminary note on the occurrence of Trypanosoma theileri in the blood of cattle. Paper 2. On the presence of Trypanosoma melophagium in the blood of Victorian sheep, and its transmission by the sheep "tick", Melophagus ovinus. J. Coun. scient. ind. Res. Aust. 3, 120-121

Uganda (1925 - 1927, 1931 - 1933 & 1948 - 1962) Annual reports of the Department of Veterinary Services (latterly Veterinary Services and Animal Industry)

Valladares, I. F. (1909) A case of Trypanosoma theileri in Madras. J. trop. vet. Sci. 4, 544-545

Van Der Maaten, M. J. & Malmquist, W. A. (1969) Elimination of Trypanosoma theileri from cell cultures by amphotericin B treatment. Am. J. vet. Res. 30, 2013-2015

Van Der Poel, P. P. (1912) Beitr"age zur Kenntnis der bei gesunden Rindern vorkommenden Trypanosomen. Aus dem Reichs - Serum - Institut zu Rotterdam. Direktor Prof. Poels. Dissertation von Bern 1912. (Abstracted in Schweizer Arch. Tierheilk. 54, 260-262

Van Saceghem, R. (1922) Trypanosoma theileri au Ruanda. Annls Soc. belge Méd. trop. 2, 113-114

Veri, -. (1920) Quoted by Curasson (1943)

Virviescas, F. (1934) Tripanosoma theileria y babesiella en la sangre de un bovino del valle del Cauca. Revta Med. vet., Bogotá 6, 898-901

Vrijburg, A. (1911) Trypanosomen bij gezonde runderen. Tijdschr. Veeartsenijk. Veeteelt 38, 353-356

Vrijburg, A. (1912) De Trypanosoma transvaliense bij hollandse runderen. Tijdschr. Veeartsenijk. Veeteelt 39, 803-812

Vrijburg, A. (1938) Trypanosomen bij van multvuur verdachte runderen. Tijdschr. Diergeneesk. 65, 512-513

Walker, P. J. (1963) Variation in the length of trypanosomes after different methods of staining. Trans. R. Soc. trop. Med. Hyg. 57, 237

Wallace, F. G. (1962) The trypanosomatid parasites of horseflies with the description of Crithidia rileyi n. sp. J. Protozool. 9, 53-58

Wallace, F. G. (1966) The trypanosomatid parasites of insects and arachnids. Expl Parasit. 18, 124-193

Watson, E. A. & Hadwen, S. (1912) Trypanosomes found in Canadian mammals. Parasitology 5, 21-26 + 2 plates

Weber (1909) Über einem nichtpathogenen Trypanosoma beim Rind. Arch. Schiffs- u. Tropenhyg. 13, Beiheft 6 p. 143

Wells, E. A. (1969) Bovine trypanosomiasis with special reference to Trypanosoma theileri. Ph. D. thesis, Univ. of Edinburgh

Wells, E. A. (1971a) Studies on Trypanosoma theileri-like trypanosomes of cattle. I. Culture and storage of isolations. Br. vet. J. 127, 466-475

Wells, E. A. (1971b) Studies on Trypanosoma theileri-like trypanosomes of cattle. II. The characteristics of infection in a single Ayrshire cow. Br. vet. J. 127, 476-484

Wells, E. A., Betancourth, A. & Page, W. A. (1970) The epidemiology of bovine trypanosomiasis in Colombia. Trop. Anim. Hlth Prod. 2, 111-125

Wells, E. A., Lumsden, W. H. R. & Hardy, G. J. C. (1965) Isolation of Trypanosoma theileri Laveran 1902, from cattle in Scotland. Nature, Lond. 206, 847

Wells, E. A., Lumsden, W. H. R. & McNeillage, G. J. C. (1968) Isolation of trypanosomes of the section Stercoraria from cattle in Nigeria and the United Kingdom. Br. vet. J. 124, 382-392

Wells, E. A., Ruiz, A. & Ochoa, R. (1968) Trypanosomiasis in Colombia. Trans. R. Soc. trop. med. Hyg. 62, 138

Wenyon, C. M. (1926) Protozoology, Vol. 1 pp. 498-501 & 507 London: Baillière, Tindall & Cox

Wester, J. J. (1911) Trypanosomen bij onze koeien. Tijdschr. Veeartsenijk. Veeteelt 38, 356-359

W. H. O. (1965) Immunology and parasitic diseases. Wld Hlth Org. techn Rep. Ser. No. 315

Wladimiroff, A. & Yakimoff, W. (1909) Bemerkung zur vorstehenden Mitteilung Wrublewskis. Zentbl. Bakt. ParasitKde 48, 164

Woo, P. T. K. (1969) The haematocrit centrifuge for the detection of trypanosomes in blood. Can. J. Zool. 47, 921-923

Woo, P., Soltys, M. A. & Gillick, A. C. (1970) Trypanosomes in cattle in southern Ontario. Can. J. comp. Med. 34, 142-147

Wrublewski, K. J. (1909) Ein Trypanosoma des Wisent von Bielowesch. Zentbl. Bakt. ParasitKde I. Orig. 48, 162-164

Wrublewski, K. J. (1912) Die Trypanosomose (Schlafkrankheit) der Wisente. Z. InfektKrankh. parasit. Krankh. Hyg. Haustiere 12, 376-384

Wyssman, E. (1935) Zur Frage der durch Trypanosoma theileri bedingten Erkrankungen beim Rind. Schweizer Arch. Tierheilk. 77, 401-415

Yakimoff, W. (1915) A propos du Trypanosoma wrublewskyi. Bull Soc. Path. exot. 8, 431-433

Yakimoff, W. L. & Kohl-Yakimoff, N. (1911a) Recherches sur les trypanosomes du genre "theileri" des bovidés en Tunisie. Première note. Présence di trypanosomes normaux dans le sang des bovidés tunisiens. Archs Inst. Pasteur, Tunis 6, 258-262

Yakimoff, W. L. & Kohl-Yakimoff, N. (1911b) Sur la présence de trypanosomes dans le sang des bovidés à Tunis. Bull. Soc. Path. exot. 4, 309

Yakimoff, W. L., Marcoff, E. N., Oulassewitsch, J. S. & Rastegaieff, E. F. (1925) Sur la repartition geographique du Trypanosoma theileri en Russie. Bull. Soc. Path. exot. 18, 57

Yakimoff, W. L. & Schokhor, W. J. (1916) A propos du Trypanosoma theileri au Turkestan Russe. Bull. Soc. Path. exot. 9, 229

Yakimov, V. L., Amanzhulov, S. A., Arbuzov, P. N. & Zhuralev, A. I. (1926) [A case of Trypanosome theileri infection in cattle in the Urals.] Russk. Zh. trop. Med. 6, 185-186

Yakimov, V. L., Nezvetaev, N. V. & Petunina, P. I. (1933) Die Blutparasiten des Zebu. Berl. tierärztl. Wschr. 49, 824-827

Yakimov, V. L. & Shokhor, N. I. (1913) [Trypanosomiasis in camels in Turkestan.] Russk. Vrach. 12, 1322

Yamada, -. (1914) Quoted by Saisawa et al. (1933)

Yang, T. -J., Hare, W. C. D. & Abt, D. A. (1967) DNA and RNA synthesis in cultures of peripheral blood mononuclear leucocytes from normal and lymphosarcomatous cows. Br. J. Haemat. 13, 855-861

Zlotnic, I. (1953) Cerebral piroplasmosis in cattle. Vet. Rec. 65, 642-643

9